The Cultural Warping of Childbirth

Improving the Outcome of Pregnancy Through Science

Doris Haire at The Bradley Method® Advanced Teacher Workshop

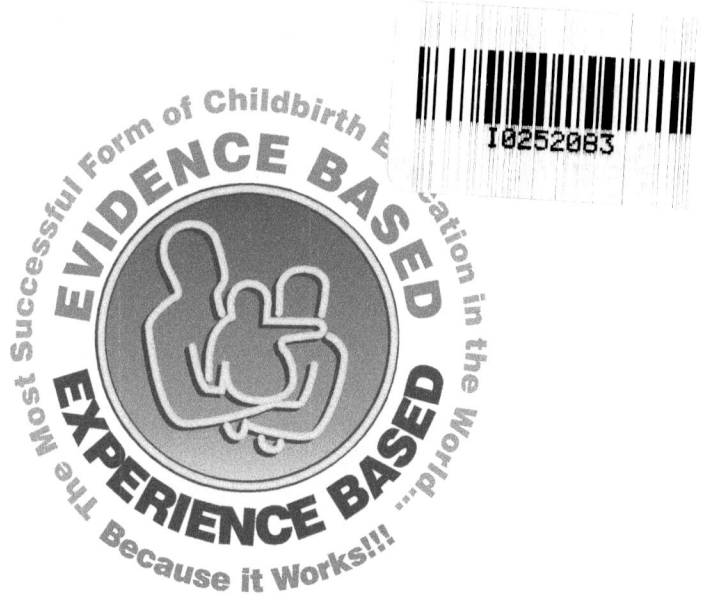

For Educational Purposes Only!

The information contained in this book is intended for educational purposes only. It does not constitute medical advice, nor is it a substitute for medical advice. You should consult a physician regarding medical diagnosis or treatment.

The Cultural Warping of Childbirth
A Special Report by
Doris Haire

Foreward

This report deserves to be read and discussed seriously by all who play a role in any phase of American maternity care. The author's analysis of the cultural warping of childbirth in the United States is thought-provoking and deserves careful consideration, whether or not the reader agrees with all of her conclusions. There is still a great deal we do not know about the consequences of various obstetrical practices and aspects of maternity care. The author's anaysis reminds us that many of our accepted practices are not supported by scientific research and appear to be rooted more in hospital and medical tradition than in human physiology. The report will be particularly useful if it causes parents and professionals alike to reevaluate American maternity pratices and their effects on the mother, the infant and the family. Its publication is timely since there is increasing evidence that parents want to become involved in those decisions which possibly will influence their future relationships with their children and with each other.

Jerold Lucey, M.D., F.A.A.P.
Professor of Pediatrics, University of Vermont
Past Chairman, Committee on Fetus and Newborn
American Academy of Pediatrics, 1966,71

About the Author

Doris Haire, AAHCC, American Academy of Husband-Coached Childbirth (The Bradley Method®) Advisor, ICEA Co-President 1970-72, former representative on U.S. Food and Drug Administration Subcommittee on Fetal Monitoring Devices. President, American Foundation for Maternal and Child Health. Founder, CEA of Metropolitan New York. Chair, National Women's Health Network, 1978-79. Author, *The Cultural Warping of Childbirth, Implementing Family-Centered Maternity Care with a Central Nursery*.

In preparing this report on *The Cultural Warping of Childbirth*, Haire, who is a medical sociologist with an honorary doctorate in medical science, visited hospitals and consulted with professionals involved in maternity care in North and South America, Western Europe, Russia, Asia, Oceania and Africa. As a medical writer she has been given the unique opportunity to attend both a school of nursing and a college of medicine as a special student in obstetrics.

THE CUTURAL WARPING OF CHILDBIRTH

WHILE Sweden, Finland and the Netherlands compete for the honor of having the lowest incidence of infant deaths per one thousand live births*, the United States continues to find itself outranked by fourteen other developed countries. (Table I).

Several explanations for our poor national infant outcome have been advanced. Some try to explain our poor standing on the grounds that our statistics are more reliable, but according to the Statistical Office of the United Nations our statistics are no more accurate than those of the other countries listed in Table I, all of which use the same U.N. standard for "live birth" without regard for gestational age or birth weight, and most of which collect their statistics on a uniform basis through their national health services. Analyses by Chase of the United States Public Health Service and more recently by Wegman, writing in Pediatrics[1] acknowledge slight variations in the collection of this data but report that, when cross checked by other statistical data, the variations do not significantly alter the statistics.

TABLE 1
INFANT MORTALITY RATES FOR LOWEST 20 COUNTRIES WITH POPULATIONS OVER 2.500,000

Country	Rate 1972	1973
Sweden	10.8	9.6
Finland	11.3	10.0
Japan	11.7	11.3
Netherlands	11.7	11.5
Denmark	12.2	11.5
Norway	11.3*	11.8*
Switzerland	13.3	13.2*
France	16.0	15.5*
Canada	17.1	15.6
German Democratic Republic	17.7	16.0
New Zealand	15.6*	16.2*
Australia	16.7	16.5*
Hong Kong	17.5	16.8*
England and Wales	17.2	16.9
Belgium	18.9	17.0*
United States	18.5	17.7
Ireland	17.8	18.0
Chechoslovakia	21.4	21.2
German Federal Republic	22.4	22.7
Israel	24.2	22.8

.. *Provisional

Source: Wegman, M.: "Annual Survey of Vital Statistics - 1974", Pediatrics, 56:960-966, December 1975.

The infant mortality rate is based on the number of infant deaths per 1,000 live births, in the first year of life. The international standard for "live birth", which is used by the United Nations, is "Any product of conception, regardless of gestational age or weight, which shows signs of heart beat, respiration, definite movement of voluntary muscles or pulsation of the umbilical cord."

In light of the fact that in most of the other listed countries there is no strong feeling of obligation to use extraordinary measures to preserve life when a live birth results in extreme prematurity, severe congenital malformation or impairment, their incidence of infant mortality should be greater than ours, not less. (Table 3).

No one will dispute the fact that socioeconomic factors play a significant role in any infant mortality statistics. However research has demonstrated that among mothers of the lower socioeconomic groups infant outcome can be substantially improved by changing the pattern of obstetrical care offered these mothers during labor and birth.[7]

There is no question that the welfare of their patients has always been the deep concern of American physicians, nurse-midwives and nurses. The unphysiological practices which have become so much a part of American obstetric care - to the point where such practices have been generally accepted as normal accompaniments of birth - appear to have gradually built up as a result of social customs and cultural patterning. But cultural patterning can be changed if mothers can be helped to recognize the importance of their accepting some inconvenience and discomfort (and at times pain) in order to achieve the best possible birth and good health for their babies.

Educating mothers for the childbearing experience and improving the quality of emotional support given to mothers during labor and birth have been clearly demonstrated to lessen or eliminate the mother's need for obstetrical medication and obstetrical intervention during labor and birth. The benefit of individualized emotional support and care during this time of stress was made evident in a report by Levy[7] who notes that during a two year medically-directed, nurse-midwifery program carried out in California, in which nurse-midwives were employed to provide complete care for normal maternity patients, the incidence of infant deaths decreased significantly.

In order to avoid the inference that it was the additional access to prenatal care alone which made the difference in infant mortality Levy compared the incidence of infant deaths among women who had had *no prenatal care at all* before, during and following the pilot program. He found that the incidence of infant mortality among mothers who had had NO prenatal care at all, but who were attended during labor and birth by a nurse-midwife, dropped significantly during the nurse-midwifery program and then almost doubled when the nurse-midwifery program ended. Across the continent the success of the California nurse-midwifery program has been essentially duplicated ...

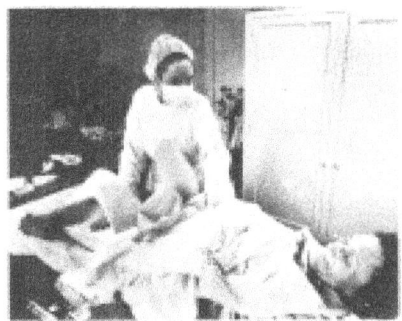

In this photograph taken by Michael Mauney for Life Magazine during a visit to the Frontier Nursing Service, the influence of European obstetrics can be seen. The student nurse-midwife checks the final contractions of a Kentucky mother as she waits patiently for the mother to give birth.

by the Frontier Nursing Service in remote Leslie County, Kentucky, one of the poorest counties in Appalachia.

Obviously we can not produce enough nurse-midwives overnight to fill the demand, but we can do much to improve our incidence of infant mortality and morbidity by maximizing the emotional support offered the childbearing woman in order that she may cope with the discomfort of labor and birth with a minimum of medication and its attendant hazards. A spokesman for the National Foundation March of Dimes recently stated that according to the most recent data, the United States leads all developed countries in the rate of infant deaths due to birth injury and respiratory distress such as postnatal asphyxia and atelectasis.

According to the National Association for Retarded Children there are now 6,000,000 retarded children and adults in the United States with a predicted annual increase of over 100,000 a year. The number of children and adults with behavioral difficulties or perceptual dysfunction resulting from minimal brain damage is an ever growing challenge to society and to the economy. While it may be easier on the conscience to blame such numbing facts solely on socio-economic factors and birth defects recent research makes it evident that obstetrical medication can play a role in our staggering incidence of neurological impairment. It may be convenient to blame our relatively poor infant outcome on a lack of facilities or inadequate government funding, but it is obvious from the research being carried out that we could effect an immediate improvement in infant outcome by changing the pattern of obstetrical care in the United States. It is time that we take a good look at the overall experience of childbirth in this country and begin to recognize how our culture has warped this experience for the majority of American mothers and their newborn infants.

I have visited hundreds of maternity hospitals throughout the world - in Great Britain, Western Europe, Russia, Asia, Australia, New Zealand, the South Pacific, the Americas and Africa. During my visits I was privileged to observe obstetric techniques and procedures and to interview physicians, professional midwives and parents in the various countries. My companion on many of my visits was Dorothea Lang, C.N.M. (Certified Nurse-Midwife), Director of Nurse-Midwifery for New York City. Miss Lang's experience as both a nurse-midwife and a former head nurse of the labor and delivery unit of the New York Cornell Medical Center made her a particularly well-qualified observer and companion. As we traveled from country to country certain patterns of care soon became evident. For one, in those countries which enjoy an incidence of infant mortality and birth trauma significantly lower than that of the United States, highly trained professional midwives are an important source of obstetrical care and family planning services for normal women, whether the births take place in the hospital or in the home. In these countries the expertise of the physician is called upon only when the expectant mother is ill during pregnancy or when labor or birth is anticipated to be, or is found to be abnormal. Under this system the high-risk mother - the one who is most likely to bear an impaired or stillborn child - has a better opportunity to obtain in-depth medical attention than is possible under ...

our existing American system of obstetrical care where the obstetrician is also called upon to play the role of midwife.

Deprivation, birth defects, prematurity and low birth weight are not unique to the United States. While it is tempting to blame our comparatively high incidence of infant mortality solely on a lack of available prenatal care and on socioeconomic factors, our observations indicate that, comparatively, the prenatal care we offer most clinic patients in the United States is not grossly inferior to that available in other developed countries. Furthermore, the diet and standard of living in many countries which have a lower incidence of infant mortality than ours would be considered inadequate by American standards.

As an example, when one compares the availability of prenatal care, the incidence of premature births, the average diet of various economic groups and the equipment available to aid in newborn infant survival in two such diverse countries as the United States and Japan, there are no major differences between the two countries. The differences lie in (a) our frequent use of prenatal and obstetrical medication, (b) our pathologically oriented management of pregnancy, labor, birth and postpartum, and (c) the predominance of artificial feeding in the United States, as opposed to Japan.

If present statistics follow the trend of recent years, an infant born in the United States is more than four times more likely to die in the first day of life than an infant born in Japan (Table 2). But survival of the birth process should not be our singular goal. For every American newborn infant who dies there are likely to be several who are neurologically damaged because the major differences in infant mortality between the United States and Japan are represented by our comparatively high incidence of infant deaths due to birth injury and respiratory distress, such as postnatal asphyxia and atelectasis (Table 3), conditions which are more likely to occur if the mother has received obstetrical medication. ...

TABLE 2
INFANT MORTALITY RATES (PER 1000 LIVE BIRTHS) IN SELECTED COUNTRIES, 1967*
Classified by Age (Day and Month).

Country	Total	0day	0d-6d.	0d.-27d.	28d.-5m.	6m.-llm.
Canada	22.0	9.0	13.6	15.2	5.3	1.5
U.S.A.	22.4	9.6	15.0	16.5	4.5	1.4
Japan	14.9	2.1	7.3	9.9	3.5	1.5
Belgium	22.9	7.3	14.0	16.0	4.9	2.1
Denmark	15.8	----	5.7	12.1	2.5	1.1
Finland	14.8	4.8	10.5	11.8	2.2	0.8
Norway	14.8	3.9	9.8	11.1	2.4	1.2
Netherlands	13.4	4.0	9.1	10.4	1.7	1.2
England & Wales	18.3	6.3	10.7	12.5	4.4	1.4
Sweden	12.9	4.4	9.4	10.5	1.5	0.8
Switzerland	17.5	7.3	12.1	13.5	2.6	1.4

TABLE 3
INFANT MORTALITY RATES (PER 1000 LIVE BIRTHS) IN SELECTED COUNTRIES, 1967*
According to Leading Causes.

	All Causes	Malignant Neoplasms	Pneumonia	Gastroenteritis	Congenital Malformation	Birth Injuries Postnatal Asphyxia and Atelectasis	Infections of the Newborn	Premature Infant	Others
Canada	22.0	0.1	1.7	0.4	4.0	4.5	0.8	7.4	3.1
U.S.A.	22.4	0.1	1.6	0.3	3.3	5.5	0.9	7.3	3.4
Japan	14.9	0.1	1.4	0.6	1.9	1.7	1.0	5.9	2.3
Belgium	22.9	0.1	0.7	0.3	4.9	3.0	1.2	8.6	4.1
Denmark	15.8	0.1	0.3	0.1	3.5	5.3	0.3	3.8	2.4
Finland	14.8	0.1	0.3	0.1	3.0	5.4	0.5	3.5	1.9
Norway	14.8	0.1	0.6	0.2	2.9	4.2	0.5	4.0	2.3
Netherlands	13.4	0.1	0.1	0.2	3.3	3.6	0.5	3.6	2.0
England & Wales	18.3	0.1	2.1	0.4	3.8	4.5	0.8	4.0	2.6
Sweden	12.9	0.1	0.3	0.1	2.7	4.3	0.3	3.7	1.4
Switzerland	17.5	0.1	0.3	0.4	3.9	4.4	0.7	5.6	2.1
New Zealand	18.0	0.1	2.1	0.3	3.7	4.6	0.7	3.4	3.1

*Information based on statistics available from the Statistical Office of the United Nations.

The better record of infant outcome in Japan is even more dramatic when one considers that, according to a recent report by the Japanese Ministry of Health, the maternal death rate due to toxemia is 5 times greater in Japan than in the United States. Whether this is due to diet or life style is not yet scientifically established.

Most American mothers do not, as yet, realize that the management of labor is even more important than the management of birth in determining how an infant will fare, not only during the first critical hours but perhaps throughout life. A poorly managed labor can result in an infant who shows no signs of respiratory distress and who scores well on the Apgar scale, while, in fact, a more scientific evaluation of the infant's condition may indicate lingering signs of oxygen deprivation in utero resulting from obstetrical medication administered to the mother.[3]

Hellman and Pritchard state that the respiratory center of the infant is highly vulnerable to sedative and anesthetic drugs administered to the mother and that such medication may jeopardize the initiation of respiration of the infant at birth. They point out that sluggish respiration is observed to some extent in the majority of infants whose mothers received sedation during labor.[4] The added burden on the newly born infant of having to detoxify indirectly acquired obstetrical medication as he adjusts to extrauterine life is the subject of abundant scientific literature in the past and present.[5-26]

An outstanding monograph entitled *"Effects of Obstetrical Medication on Fetus and Newborn,"* June, 1970, published by the Society for Research in Child Development, makes it evident that we can no longer assume that the apparent recovery of an asphyxiated infant after successful resuscitation is a guarantee that the infant has come through unharmed.[6] (This monograph should be required reading for all obstetrical personnel). A baby with a heartbeat after cardiac massage may appear to be recovered but, in fact, may be irreversibly brain damaged.[8] Virtually all obstetrical medications- nausea remedies, diuretics, sedatives, muscle relaxants, analgesics, regional anesthesia and general anesthetics-tend to rapidly cross the placenta and alter the fetal environment as they enter the circulatory system of the unborn infant within seconds or minutes of administration to the mother.[5-26] As Dr. Virginia Apgar bluntly puts it, the placenta is not a barrier but a "bloody sieve."

If prolapse of the umbilical cord or premature separation of the placenta occurs during labor the fetus is compromised. If obstetrical medication is administered to the mother during labor and either of these conditions occurs this compounds the danger to the unborn infant. No one can guarantee the mother that such conditions will not occur.

While respiratory distress is one of the more obvious hazards of obstetrical medication, the more subtle effects of such medications are now being noted. Sedatives containing barbiturates administered to the mother during labor have been shown to adversely affect the infant's suckling reflexes for 4 or 5 days after birth.[9,10] The prolonged effects of some commonly used obstetrical medications, such as meperidine (Demerol), have been detected in the infant several weeks after birth.[23]

Regional anesthesias appear to be an improvement over general anesthesia but research indicates that even in the most dedicated hands regional anesthesias can compromise the mother and her infant. All regional anesthesias, including pudendal block, tend to alter the fetal environment and to inhibit the mother's ability to push her baby down the birth canal[24] which in turn, tends to increase the need for fundal pressure, uterine stimulants and forceps extraction -conditions which should be avoided if possible in the best interests of the child.[74,60,29] L. Stanley James, Chairman of the Committee on Fetus and Newborn of the American Academy of Pediatrics, cautions, "Regional techniques are gaining popularity but they are not without problems." He points out that it is difficult to give spinal anesthesia - caudal, epidural, or saddle block - without any change in maternal blood pressure, and that even if pressure is restored by the use of vasopressors there is no assurance that regional circulation through the uterus remains normal.[15]

Because he must fill the role of both obstetrician and midwife, the overburdened American obstetrician frequently manages his maternity patient's labor by telephone and arrives at the hospital shortly before a birth is anticipated. This type of management must depend on reports from the mother's labor attendant, who may or may not have had specialized training in evaluating the effects of labor and obstetrical medication on both the mother and her unborn infant. But in countries which enjoy a lower incidence of infant mortality than ours it is the hospital-assigned, professional midwife who manages the prenatal care, labor, ...

birth and postpartum care of the normal mother and the care of the normal newborn infant. The professional midwife receives special training in maintaining the delicate physiologic balance between mother and child during labor and birth, and is trained to recognize conditions which require the medical expertise of the physician.

Because the professional midwife also is involved in the postpartum care of the infant, and not just labor and delivery, she is fully aware of the importance of providing individualized and skillful emotional support for the laboring mother as a means of reducing or eliminating the mother's need for obstetrical medication, with its possible narcotizing effect on the fetus and newborn infant.

The active encouragement of breastfeeding by the professional midwife also appears to affect the incidence of infant mortality in the various countries, for in those countries such as Sweden, the Netherlands and Japan, where breastfeeding is still the predominant pattern of initial infant feeding, the incidence of infant mortality is significantly lower than in those countries where artificial feeding is the predominant initial form of infant feeding. It is interesting to note that in those older age categories, when the customary times for weaning occur, such countries as Sweden, the Netherlands and Japan begin to lose their statistical advantages (Table 2).

Unfortunately, the American tendency to warp the birth experience, distorting it into a pathological event, rather than a physiological one, for the normal childbearing woman is no longer peculiar to just the United States. In my visits to hospitals in various countries I was distressed to find that some physicians, anxious to impress their colleagues with their "Americanized" techniques, have unfortunately adopted many of our obstetrical practices without stopping to question their scientific or social merit.

Few American babies are born today as nature intended them to be. Among the 55,000 children included in the American Collaborative Perinatal Study carried out by the National Institute of Neurological Diseases and Stroke, there was no apparent effort made to include a control group of normal mothers who were educated to cope with the discomfort of childbirth without the use of medication. With rare exception, those mothers in the Collaborative Study who did not receive obstetrical medication were those who had a precipitous labor or those whose unborn child showed signs of fetal distress which precluded the use of obstetrical medication.

Although there is a tendency to think of paracervical and pudendal block anesthesia as relatively harmless, research indicates that they too can compromise the fetus and newborn infant.[18, 24, 26] Rosefsky and Petersiel noted a drop in fetal heart rate in almost half of a group of 93 mothers who were observed after receiving paracervical block anesthesia. In another series the incidence of infant depression and Apgar scores of 6 or less was almost 3 times greater among those infants whose mothers had received paracervical block than among the controls. The fetal hazards of depression with occasional death associated with paracervical block have been clearly demonstrated.[27] Transient fetal bradycardia may appear to be relatively harmless but an abnormal drop in fetal heart rate usually indicates a decrease in the oxygen saturation of the fetus.[30, 31] How much depletion of oxygen can be sustained by a given fetus or newborn infant before neurological damage occurs ...

may not be recognized for several years, for the effect of even a relatively small decrease in oxygen saturation of the fetus and newborn has yet to be assessed. It is ironic that transient fetal bradycardia is taken so lightly, for no one would purposely inject medication or apply a device to a newborn infant which would possibly decrease his oxygen supply for even a few minutes without grave cause.

The relaxed attitude in the past toward the use of obstetrical medication was not due to a lack of concern for the fetus and newborn infant but to an unawareness of the problem. However, newer scientific methods of evaluating the immediate and prolonged effects on the fetus and newborn infant of obstetrical medications and many of our common obstetrical practices now make it evident that they do, in fact, tend to alter the normal fetal and infant environment. The effect of ...

METHOD OF SCORING FOR APGAR SCORE

Sixty seconds and again at five minutes after the complete birth of the infant (disregarding the cord and placenta) the following five objective signs are evaluated and each given a score of 0, 1, or 2. A score of 10 indicates an infant is in the best possible condition. Infants with scores of 5 to 10 usually need no immediate treatment. A score of 4 or below indicates the need for prompt diagnosis and treatment.

Sign	0	1	2	1 Min. Score	5 Min. Score
Heart Rate	Absent	Slow (Below 100)	Over 100		
Respiratory Effort	Absent	Slow Irregular	Good Crying		
Muscle Tone	Limp	Some Flexion of Extremities	Active Motion		
Reflex Irritability: Response to Catheter in Nostril	No Response	Grimace	Cough or Sneeze		
Color	Blue, Pale	Body Pink. Extremities Blue	Completely Pink *		

*American professionals are frequently amazed to see the consistency with which Scandinavian and Dutch newborn infants "pink up" to the very tips of their fingers and toes a few seconds after being born.

minimal brain damage on the child's personality and his ability to learn and to cope with our complex society is only now beginning to be fully understood.[8] Research by Lewis indicates that infants who were rated between 7 to 9 on the Apgar scale at birth were significantly less attentive than were those infants rated 10, and that the difference, in general, held true over the first year of life.[16] It is not unlikely that unnecessary alterations in the normal fetal environment may play a role in the incidence of neurological impairment and infant mortality in the United States. Infant resuscitation, other than routine suctioning, is rarely needed in countries such as Sweden, the Netherlands and Japan, where the skillful psychological management of labor usually precludes the need for obstetrical medication. In contrast, in those European countries, such as Belgium, where the overall pattern of obstetrical care is similar to our own the incidence of infant mortality also approaches our own.

Obviously there will always be medical indications which dictate the use of various obstetrical procedures, but to apply the following American practices and procedures routinely to the vast majority of mothers who are capable of giving birth without complication is to create added stress which is not in the best interests of either the mother or her newborn infant.

Let us take a close look at our infant mortality statistics and then at some of our common obstetrical practices from early pregnancy to postpartum which have served to warp and distort the childbearing experience in the United States. While not all of the practices below affect infant mortality it is equally apparent that they do not contribute to the reduction of infant morbidity or ...

mortality and therefore should be reevaluated.

❏ *After you have read each section below, check the appropriate box if the obstetrical care in your community includes the practice discussed.*

The total number of check marks that you record will provide some idea as to how far obstetric practices in your community have digressed from normal physiological childbirth.

❏ **Withholding Information on the Disadvantages of Obstetrical Medication**

Ignorance of the possible hazards of obstetrical medication appears to encourage the misuse and abuse of obstetrical medication, for in those countries where mothers are not told routinely of the possible disadvantages of obstetrical medication to themselves or to their babies the use of such medication is on the increase.

There is no research or evidence which indicates that mothers will be emotionally damaged if they are advised, prior to birth, that obstetrical medication may be to the disadvantage of their newborn infants. Offering the mother accurate, printed information (adapted from that which appears in the package insert of every obstetrical medication) on the relative safety and hazards of commonly used obstetrical medications and practices, prior to her confinement, may seem a nuisance, but such a precaution helps to protect the hospital, physician or professional midwife from legal liability resulting from the mother's uninformed consent and allows the mother to share in the responsibility for her own well-being and that of her child in utero. To withhold information as to the possible complications of obstetrical medication is to delude the mother into assuming that there are no risks involved.

We must keep in mind that it is the mother who must ultimately bear the major emotional burden of a damaged or impaired child, even if that child is institutionalized. Under normal conditions no one should usurp the mother's prerogative by placing her unborn or newborn infant at a possible disadvantage without her informed consent. As the public becomes more aware of the possible effects of obstetrical practices on infant outcome, failure to disclose or inform the mother of the possible adverse consequences of some of the obstetrical practices discussed herein may become the basis of legal liability if or when those adverse consequences occur.[32]

❏ **Ambivalent Prenatal Counseling on Breast-Feeding**

In most of the countries of the world breast-feeding is actively encouraged during the prenatal counseling and during the mother's hospital confinement. Breast-feeding is particularly encouraged if birth is premature. If an infant is too premature or ill to suckle his mother's breasts the mother is frequently asked to return to the hospital in order to express her milk in the presence of her baby, since the closeness tends to increase the mother's production of milk. In contrast, most American mothers are merely asked prenatally, to state their preference for breast feeding or bottle feeding, without being offered any information as to the relative benefits of breast-feeding to their babies. Once the mother has stated her preference to bottle-feed, little or no effort is made to suggest to her the advantages of breast-feeding. Yet the incidence of allergy among formula-fed infants is steadily on the rise in the United States.[33,34]

While not all of the protective mechanisms of breast milk are ...

understood, many scientists have demonstrated that there is signifi-cantly less incidence of illness among children who are breast-fed.[35,36] A survey of over 3,000 children living in a housing project in England (post-penicillin) showed that the death rate was 9 times greater among children who were artificially fed from birth. All of the children in the project received their health care from the same doctors and nurses. Yet among those children who were breast-fed there was significantly less incidence of common colds, bronchitis, pneumonia, eczema, asthma, hayfever, colic, gastroenteritis, otitis media, mastoid, whooping cough, measles, german measles, and scarlet fever.[37] Colostrum and breast milk contain antibodies against three strains of polio, Coxsackie B. Virus, two types of colon bacilli which can cause fatal infant diarrhea,[38] pathogenic strains of E coli., and gram-negative infections.[39,41]

Diseases resulting from malab-sorption, such as celiac syndrome,[42,43] and sudden infant death syndrome (SIDS) rarely occur among completely breast-fed babies." Unfortunately there are too few breast-fed infants in the high incidence SIDS study areas to make up an adequate number of breast-fed controls.[45] Newborn infants who are breast-fed excrete more strontium than is ingested in breast-milk whereas bottlefed infants accumulate strontium.[46,47]

There are now indications that the protective effects of breast milk may go far beyond the weaning period. Various researchers suggest that there is less incidence of dental caries,[48] orthodontic disproportion and orofacial dental deformities,[49,50] premature atherosclerosis,[5,52] and ulcerative colitis among young people and adults who were initially breast-fed.[53] One can only wonder about the future incidence of ulcerative colitis among adults whose initial food was foreign protein, fed at a temperature 25° below the temperature of breast milk, an infant's normal, species specific food. Research is strongly supportive of the use of breast milk for the premature infant.[5,40,54,55] Mothers who breast-feed were noted by Paffenberger to show a decreased susceptibility to delayed postpartum hemorrhage.[56] In light of the abundant research showing the medical value of breast-feeding it would seem that a statement such as, "One is just as good as another" can hardly be applied to the initial form of feeding of a newborn infant. ...

For additional information and references on this subject read, "The Nurse's Contribution to Successful BreastFeeding," prepared by the author.[57]

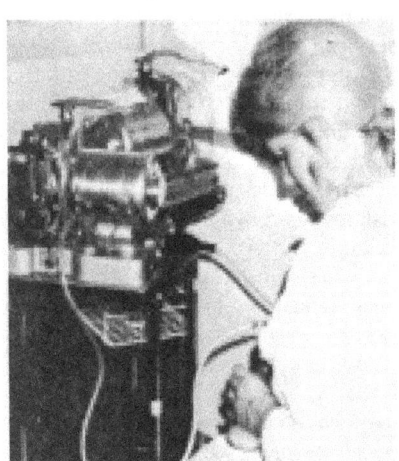

To provide sufficient breast milk for premature and ill infants Swedish mothers are asked to contribute excess breast milk during their postpartum stay.

❏ **Permitting the Mother to Face Childbirth Uninformed of Ways in which She Can Help Herself to Cope with the Discomfort of Labor and Birth**

All mothers should be offered the opportunity to be physically and emotionally prepared to cope with the discomfort of childbirth because circumstances frequently preclude the use of obstetrical medication, even if the mother requests it. Dr. Charles Flowers, former Chairman of the Committee on Obstetric Analgesia and Anesthesia of the American College of Obstetricians and Gynecologists, states "Gymnastics are not necessary in the preparation of the patient for childbirth but the ability of a person to know what to do and how to relax and how to breathe during labor is of fundamental importance." [13]

A well-controlled research program by Enkin[58] of Canada demonstrated that mothers who were prepared for the possibility of effectively participating in the birth process tended to experience significantly shorter labors, to require less medication and less obstetrical intervention and to remember the experience of birth more favorably than did those mothers who were motivated to ask to be prepared to cope with childbirth but could not be accommodated in classes.

According to Dr. Pierre Vellay, a pioneer in childbirth education, the ability to relax is the key to pain relief during labor and birth and the breathing patterns act as a distraction from painful stimuli. Experience in several countries indicates that the type of controlled breathing patterns, either chest or abdominal, taught in class or in the labor room is relatively unimportant since it is the mother's intense concentration on the controlled breathing patterns, and not the breathing patterns in themselves, which

makes her less aware of the discomfort or pain of her contractions.

The psychoprophylactic method of childbirth training, developed and still used successfully in Russia, involves no controlled breathing patterns. The recent deemphasis on breathing patterns will help to avoid hyperventilation (according to McCance hyperventilation rarely occurs in animals!) and will help to bring childbirth educators into greater agreement.

❏ **Requiring All Normal Women to Give Birth in the Hospital**

There is ample evidence in the Netherlands and in Chicago (Chicago Maternity Center) to demonstrate that normal women who have received adequate prenatal care can safely give birth at home if a proper system is developed for home deliveries. Over half of the mothers in the Netherlands give birth at home with the assistance of a professional midwife and a maternity aide. The comparatively low incidence of infant deaths and birth trauma in the Netherlands, a country of diverse ethnic composition and intermarriage, is evidence of the comparative safety of a properly developed home delivery service.

Dutch obstetricians point out that when the labor of a normal woman is unhurried and allowed to progress normally unexpected emergencies rarely occur.They also point out that the small risk involved in a Dutch home delivery is more than offset by the increased hazards resulting from the use of obstetrical ...

medication and obstetrical tampering which are more likely to occur in a hospital environment, especially in countries where professionals have had little or no exposure to normal labor and birth in a home environment during their training. We cannot justify deprecating a system of care which rarely produces a newborn infant with an Apgar score less than 9 when we in the U.S. have a predicted yearly increase of more than 100,000 retarded infants. If the increasing American trend toward home deliveries is to be contained, it is imperative that an effort be made to make birth in the hospital as normal, as homelike and as inexpensive as possible.

❑ **Elective Induction of Labor**

The elective induction of labor (where there is no clear medical indication) appears to be an American idiosyncrasy which is frowned upon in other developed countries. In discussing elective induction of labor in *Williams Obstetrics. 14th Ed.*, Hellman and Pritchard caution that the conveniences of elective induction are not without the attendant hazards of prematurity, prolonged latent period with intrapartum infection, and prolapse of the umbilical cord. They report that studies involving almost 10,000 elective inductions indicate that perinatal deaths due to premature elective inductions occur despite efforts to comply with specific criteria.[4]

In reviewing the results of 3,324 elective inductions of labor at the University of Pennsylvania Hospital, Fields stresses the importance of caution in the selection of candidates for elective induction. He states, "Amniotomy carries with it the risk of injury to the mother or fetus and displacement of the presenting part, resulting in malposition, prolapsed cord, prolonged latent period and infection. The hazards of the use of oxytocin in labor are related directly to the dose for a given individual. Overdosage results in uterine spasm with possible separation of the placenta, tumultuous labor, amniotic fluid embolus, afibrinogenemia, lacerations of the cervix and birth canal, postpartum hemorrhage and uterine rupture. There may be water intoxication due to the antidiuretic effect of oxytocin. There may be fetal distress due to anoxia and intracranial hemorrhage, and trauma may result from tumultuous uterine contractions. Fetal and/or maternal mortality are, of course, ever-present dangers." [59,60]

The elective induction of labor has been found to almost double the incidence of fetomaternal transfusion and its attendant hazards.[61] But perhaps the least appreciated problem of elective induction is the fact that the abrupt onset of artificially induced labor tends to make it extremely difficult for even the well prepared mother to tolerate the discomfort of the intensified ontractions without the aid of obstetrical medication. When the onset of labor occurs spontaneously the normal, gradual increase in contraction length and intensity appears to provoke in the mother an accompanying tolerance for discomfort or pain.

Since the British Perinatal Hazards Study[62] found no increase in perinatal mortality or impairment of learning ability at age 7 among full term infants, unless gestation had extended beyond 42 weeks, there would appear to be no medical justification for subjecting a mother or her baby to the possible hazards of elective induction in order to terminate the pregnancy prior to 42 weeks gestation. The elective induction of ...

labor, when there is no specific medical indication, could be considered obstetrical interference in the normal physiology of childbirth and may leave the participating accoucheur legally vulnerable unless the mother is offered accurate information as to the possible hazards of elective induction of labor.

❏ **Separating the Mother from Familial Support During Labor and Birth**

Research indicates that fear adversely affects uterine motility and blood flow[63] and yet many American mothers are routinely separated from a family member or close friend at this time of emotional crisis. Mice whose labors were environmentally disturbed experienced significantly longer labors, as much as 72% longer under some conditions, and gave birth to 54% more dead pups than did the mice in the control group. Newton cautions that the human mammal, which has a more highly developed nervous system than the mouse, may be equally sensitive to environmental disturbances in labor.[98] In most developed countries, other than the United States and the Eastern European countries, mothers are encouraged to walk about or to sit and chat with a family member or supportive person in what is called an "Early Labor Lounge." This lounge is usually located near but outside the labor-delivery area in order to provide a more relaxed atmosphere during much of labor. The mother is taken to the labor-delivery area to be checked periodically, then allowed to return to the labor lounge for as long as she likes or until her membranes have ruptured.

The rapid acceptance by professionals of permitting the mother to be emotionally supported by a family member during birth is perhaps the most dramatic change in obstetrical care throughout the developed countries. However, in some countries where multiple bed delivery rooms are prevalent, such as in the eastern European countries and Asia, husbands are usually excluded.

❏ **Confining the Normal Laboring Woman to Bed**

In virtually all countries except the United States, a woman in labor is routinely encouraged to walk about during labor for as long as she wishes or until her membranes have ruptured. Such activity is considered to facilitate labor by distracting the mother's attention from the discomfort or pain of her contractions and to encourage a more rapid engagement of the fetal head. In America, where drugs are frequently administered either orally or parenterally to laboring mothers, such ambulation is discouraged - not only for the patient's safety but also to avoid possible legal complications in the event of an accident.

The disadvantages to the fetus resulting from the mother's lying in a recumbent ...

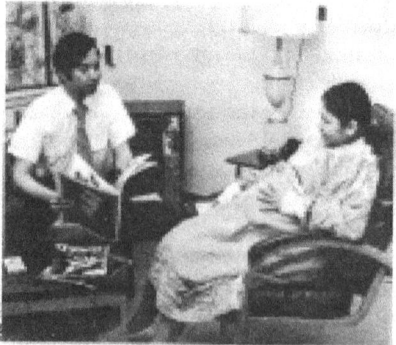

In many American Hospitals the European influence can now be seen. These parents-to-be relax in the Early Labor Lounge.

position during labor have been recognized for several years.[15,64] It is not unlikely that research will eventually find that the peasant woman who labored in the fields up until the moment of birth may have been well served by this physical activity.

❏ Shaving the Birth Area

Research involving 7,600 mothers has demonstrated that the practice of shaving the perineum and pubis does not reduce the incidence of infection. In fact, the incidence of infection was slightly higher among those mothers who were shaved.[65,66] Yet this procedure, which tends to create apprehension in laboring women, is still carried out routinely in most American hospitals. Clipping the perineal or pudendal hair closely with
surgical scissors is far less disturbing to the mother and is less likely to result in infection caused by razor abrasions.

❏ Withholding Food and Drink from the Normal Unmedicated Woman in Labor

The effect on the fetus of depriving a mother of food and drink for many hours, as is the custom in the United States, has not been sufficiently investigated. Intravenous feeding, as a substitute for light eating, only adds to the pathologic environment of an American hospital birth. In most developed countries one of the incentives for an expectant mother to take advantage of prenatal care is the fact that she will be allowed to eat and drink lightly during labor only if her prenatal examinations show her to be normal. Since anesthesia is not routinely administered during childbirth light eating and drinking has not been found to increase the incidence of maternal morbidity or mortality in these countries.

The inhalation of gastric fluid by itself can be hazardous to the anesthetized mother. Therefore, to avoid this hazard obstetricians in most countries require that the mother's stomach be emptied or special precautions be taken if for any reason she must be anesthetized for delivery.

❏ Professional Dependence on Technology and Pharmacological Methods of Pain Relief

Most of the world's mothers receive little or no drugs during pregnancy, labor or birth. The constant emotional support provided the laboring woman in other countries by the nurse-midwife, and often by her husband, appears to greatly improve the mother's tolerance for discomfort. In contrast, the American labor room nurse is frequently assigned to look after several women in labor, all or most of whom have had no preparation to cope with the discomfort or pain of childbearing. Under the circumstances drugs, rather than skillful emotional support, are employed to relieve the mother's apprehension and discomfort (and perhaps to assuage the harried labor
attendant's feeling of inadequacy). ...

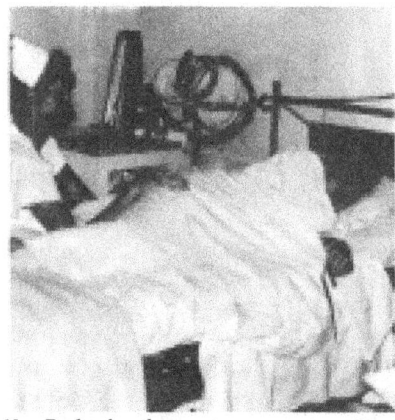

New Zealand mother receives constant emotional support during labor from nurse-midwife.

The fallacy of depending on the stethoscope to accurately monitor the effects of obstetrical medication on the well-being of the fetus has been demonstrated by Hon.[30,31] While electronic fetal monitoring is more accurate, the fact that some monitoring devices require that a mother's membranes be ruptured and that the electrode penetrate the skin of the fetal scalp creates possible hazards of its own. Therefore, obstetrical management which reduces the need for such monitoring is advisable.

Many professionals contend that a "good experience" for the mother is of paramount importance in childbearing. They tend to forget that, for the vast majority of mothers, a healthy undamaged baby is the far more important objective of childbirth. The two objectives are not always compatible. Human maternal response has not been demonstrated to be adversely altered by a stressful, unmedicated labor if the mother has been prepared for the experience of birth. To expose a mother to the possibility of a lifetime of heartache or anguish in order to insure her a few hours of comfort is misguided kindness, for while analgesia and anesthesia for the laboring woman may be the easier route for the nurse, midwife or physician, the price of a narcotized mother may be a narcotized or damaged newborn infant whose ultimate potential for learning is forever diminished.

❏ Chemical Stimulation of Labor

Oxytocic agents are frequently administered to American mothers in order to intensify artificially the frequency and/or the strength of the mother's contractions, as a means of shortening the mother's labor. While chemical stimulation is sometimes medically indicated, often it is undertaken to satisfy the American propensity for efficiency and speed. Hon suggests that the overenthusiastic use of oxytocic stimulants sometimes results in alterations in the normal fetal heart rate.[30] Fields points out that the possible hazards inherent in elective induction are also possible in artificially stimulated labor unless the mother and fetus are carefully monitored.[59,60]

The British Perinatal Study appears to consider 24 hours as an outside limit for the first stage of labor, with a second stage of 2 or 3 hours or more. The average labor is about 13 hours for a primipara and about 7 1/2 hours for a multipara." Shortening the phases of normal labor when there is no sign of fetal distress has not been shown to improve infant outcome. Little is known of the long term effects of artificially stimulating labor contractions. During a contraction the unborn child normally receives less oxygen. The gradual buildup of intensity, which occurs when the onset
of labor is allowed to occur spon- ...

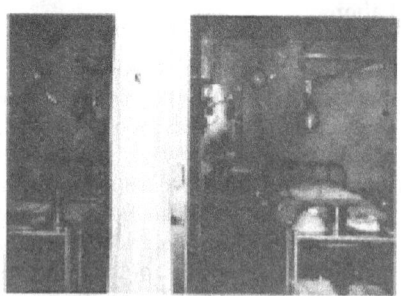

Although the small Labor-Delivery-Recovery Rooms adjacent to the infant examining area at the University of Amsterdam maternity hospital would be cramped for an "American style" delivery. births here are accomplished with quiet dignity. Emotional support and encouragement provided by the professional midwife and the husband serve as effective psychological analgesic for the mother.

taneously and to proceed without chemical stimulation, appears likely to be a protective mechanism that is best left unaltered unless there is a clear medical indication for the artificial stimulation of labor.

❏ Moving the Normal Mother to a Delivery Room for Birth

Most of the world's mothers, in both developed and developing countries, give birth in the same bed in the same hospital room in which they have labored. Since most European labor-delivery beds do not have adjustable backrests mothers are supported into a semi-sitting position for birth by their husbands or a midwife. The midwife assists the mother, and if necessary, performs an episiotomy from the side of the bed, rather from the end of the bed. The suturing of an episiotomy is done from the side of the bed, or the bed may be "broken."

American nurse-midwives, especially those who have been trained abroad, are now beginning to permit American mothers the same privilege. This may seem innovative to many Americans until we realize that there is no research or evidence which indicates that a normal, ...

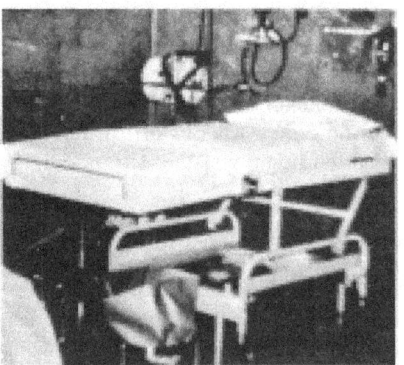

Labor-delivery bed in Sydney. Australia is comfortable for birth in either a semi-sitting or left lateral position.

essentially unmedicated mother should be required to give birth in a delivery room, rather than in a labor room which is equipped with portable or permanent sources of oxygen, suction and high intensity lighting. The pathological environment of the modern American delivery room is not conducive to a relaxed, normal childbirth experience. The low temperature of the average delivery room has in the past been more suitable for the staff than for the infant. The American Academy of Pediatrics, acting as the infant's advocate, now recommends that the temperature of the delivery room should be maintained between 71.6 and 75.2° F.[67]

❏ Delaying Birth Until the Physician Arrives

Because of the increased likelihood of resultant brain damage to the infant the practice of delaying birth by anesthesia or physical restraint until the physician arrives to deliver the infant is frowned upon in most countries. Yet the practice still occurs occasionally in the United States and in countries where hospital assigned midwives do not routinely ...

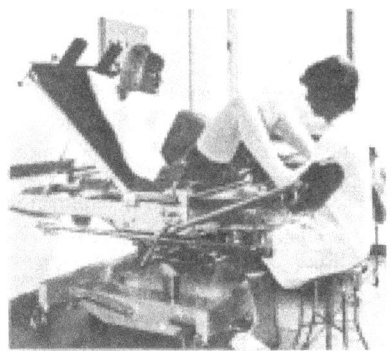

Labor-delivery bed in Stockholm. Sweden.

manage the labor and delivery of normal mothers. One of the benefits of husband attended deliveries noted by many chiefs of American obstetrical departments is the tendency for obstetrical coverage by attending physicians to immediately improve.

❏ Requiring the Mother to Assume the Lithotomy Position for Birth

Some contend that the low incidence of spontaneous births among American mothers is due to the disparity in the size between the parents, resulting from the differences in their ethnic background. However, there is gathering scientific evidence that the unphysiological lithotomy position (back flat, with knees drawn up and spread wide apart by "stirrups") which is preferred by most American physicians because it is more convenient for the accoucheur, tends to alter the normal fetal environment and obstruct the normal process of childbearing, making spontaneous birth more difficult or impossible. ...

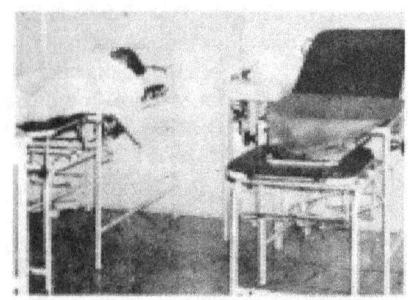

Recovering mother in a Russian maternity hospital. The undraped table on the right is in the position used for delivery.

The lithotomy and dorsal positions tend to:

1. adversely affect the mother's blood pressure, cardiac return and pulmonary ventiiation. [13,15,68]
2. decrease the normal intensity of the contractions.[68, 69, 70]
3. inhibit the mother's voluntary efforts to push her baby out spontaneously [68],[69,71] which, in turn, increases the need for fundal pressure or forceps and increases the traction necessary for a forceps extraction.
4. inhibit the spontaneous expulsion of the placenta [71] which in turn, increases the need for cord traction, forced expression or manual removal of the placenta [79] - procedures which significantly increase the incidence of fetomaternal. hemorrhage.[61]
5. increase the need for episiotomy because of the increased tension on the pelvic floor and the stretching of the perineal tissue." The normal separation of the feet for natural expulsion is about 15 to 16 inches, or 38 to 41 centimeters, which is far less separation than is allowed by the average American delivery table stirrups.

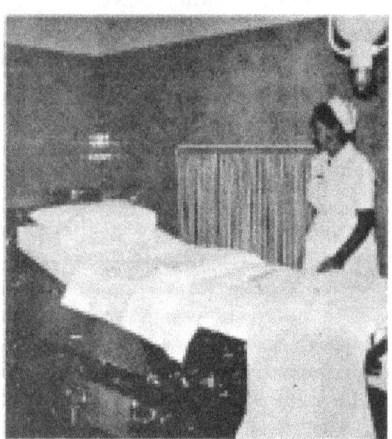

Swiss midwife stands beside adjustable labor-delivery bed.

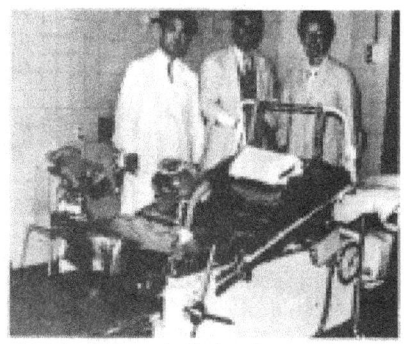

This labor-delivery bed being shown to the author at the University of Tokyo bridges two worlds. The bed adjusts to a chair-like position for birth, but also has foot stirrups if needed.

Australian, Russian and American research bears out the clinical experience of European physicians and midwives - that when mothers are supported to a semi-sitting position for birth, with their feet supported by the lower section of the labor-delivery bed (see cut), mothers tend to push more effectively, appear to need less pain relief, are more likely to want to be conscious for birth and are less likely to need an episiotomy.[68,71]

The fact that the extended delivery table or bed spares the mother the common but often unspoken fear of involuntarily expelling her baby onto the floor before the doctor or midwife is ready to receive the infant, or the fear that the accoucheur might accidentally drop her baby may inhibit the mother's ability to relax her perineum during the second stage of labor.

The increased efficiency of the semi-sitting position, combined with a minimum use of medication for birth, is evidenced by the fact that the combined use of both forceps and the vacuum extractor rarely exceeds 4% to 5% of all births in the Netherlands, as compared to an incidence of 65% in many American hospitals. (Cesarean section occurs in approximately 1.5% of all Dutch births.)

These differences are even more striking when one considers that in modern Holland, which has a, population almost as heterogeneous as our own, the average pelvic measurements of the Dutch mother and the average circumference of her baby's head are the same as those of their American counterparts.

Manual removal of the placenta occurs in approximately.6% of all Dutch births despite the fact that oxytocin is not administered to mothers routinely. Although the author knows of no specific research which verifies the incidence, clinical experience in the United States suggests that mothers who give birth in the semi-sitting position, with their legs resting on the bed, are less likely to sustain postpartum backache and fracture of the coccyx. A scientific investigation is long overdue.

❏ **The Routine Use of Regional or General Anesthesia for Delivery**

In light of the current shortage of qualified anesthetists and anesthesiologists and the frequent scientific papers now being published on the possible hazards resulting from the use of regional and general anesthesia it would seem prudent to make every effort to prepare ...

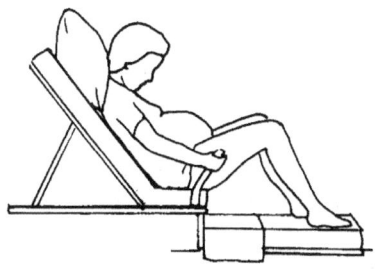

American delivery table adapted for physiological position for birth

the mother physically and mentally to cope with the sensations and discomfort of birth in order to avoid the use of such medicaments. Regional and general anesthesia not only tend to adversely affect fetal environment pharmacologically, which has been discussed previously herein, but their use also increases the need for obstetrical intervention in the normal process of birth since both types of anesthesia tend to prolong labor.[4] Johnson points out that peridural and spinal anesthesia significantly increase the incidence of midforceps delivery and its attendant hazards.[24] Pudendal block anesthesia not only tends to interfere with the mother's ability to effectively push her baby down the birth canal due to the blocking of the afferent path of the pushing reflex but
also appears to interfere with the mother's normal protective reflexes, thus making "an explosive" birth and perineal damage more likely to occur. While there are exceptions, the use of regional and general anesthesia usually dictates that:

1. the mother must be restricted from eating or drinking from the onset of labor,
2. the mother's uterine contractions must frequently be pharmacologically stimulated,
3. the mother must be moved to a delivery room which is equipped for obstetrical emergencies (obstetrical medication tends to increase the need for resuscitative measures for the infant),
4. the mother must be placed in the lithotomy position for delivery since she will not be in control of her legs,
5. fundal pressure and/or the use of forceps and an episiotomy will be needed to facilitate the delivery of the infant,
6. the infant's umbilical cord will be clamped early to facilitate immediate resuscitative measures for the infant and to shorten the infant's accumulation of obstetrical medication,
7. fundal pressure or manipulation, cord traction, pharmacological stimulation of contractions or manual removal of the placenta be employed in order to facilitate the prompt delivery of the placenta to prevent maternal hemorrhage.

❏ Fundal Pressure to Facilitate Delivery

Cooperman cites the past work of Pennoyer as he points out that the application of pressure on the fundus during delivery has been shown to depress oxygen saturation in the newborn infant.[74]
The use of obstetrical medications which tend to precipitate the use of fundal pressure should be avoided in the best interests of the mother and her infant.

❏ The Routine Use of Forceps for Delivery

There is no scientific justification for the routine application of forceps for delivery. The incidence of delivery by forceps and vacuum extractor, combined, rarely rises above 5% in countries where mothers actively participate in the births of their babies. In contrast, as mentioned previously, the incidence of forceps extraction frequently rises to as high as 65% in some American hospitals. Research in Europe, where there are more natural births to serve as controls, has demonstrated that, when forceps are used for delivery in order to relieve maternal distress, those infants so delivered are more likely to sustain intracranial hemorrhage and damage to the facial nerve or the brachial plexus.[29] There are obviously times whe indications of fetal distress dictate the use of forceps to facilitate the safe delivery of an infant but there is no scientific support for the routine application of forceps during birth.[62]

❏ Routine Episiotomy

There is no research or evidence to indicate that routine episiotomy (a surgical incision to enlarge the vaginal orifice) reduces the incidence of pelvic relaxation (structural damage to the pelvic floor musculature) in the mother. Nor is there any research or evidence that routine episiotomy reduces neurological impairment in the child who has shown no signs of fetal distress or that the procedure helps to maintain subsequent male or female sexual response.

Pelvic Relaxation: The incidence of pelvic floor relaxation appears to be on the decline throughout the world, even in those countries where episiotomy is still comparatively rare. The contention that the modern washing machine has been more effective in reducing pelvic relaxation among American mothers than has routine episiotomy is given some credence by the fact that in areas of the United States where life is still hard for the woman pelvic relaxation appears in white women who have never borne children. Interviews with gynecologists in many countries suggest that the incidence of pelvic relaxation is strongly influenced by genetics. The condition, although comparatively rare in both Fiji and Kenya, occurs more frequently among Indian women in those countries than among black women, although the living habits and fertility rate of both groups of women are much the same. Whether a resistance to pelvic relaxation is due to diet, physical activity, practices or position used during birth or any other factor is not clear. The fact remains, however, that susceptibility to pelvic relaxation appears to be a genetic weakness which has not been shown to be eliminated or reduced by routine episiotomy.

Neurological Impairment: Shortening the second stage of labor by performing an episiotomy when there is no sign of fetal distress has not been shown to be beneficial to the infant. The scientific evaluation of 17,000 children, born in one week's time and followed for 7 years in Great Britain, indicates that a second stage of labor lasting as long as two and one-half hours does not increase the incidence of neurological impairment of the full-term, average-for-gestational age infant who shows no signs of fetal distress.[62]

Sexual Response: In developed countries where episiotomy is comparatively rare the physiotherapist is considered an important member of the obstetrical team - before, as well as after birth. The physiotherapist is responsible for seeing that each mother begins exercises the day following birth which will help to restore the normal elasticity and tone of the mother's perineal and abdominal muscles. In countries where every effort is made to avoid the need for an episiotomy, interviews with both parents and professionals indicate that an intact perineum which is strengthened by postpartum exercises is more apt to result in both male and female sexual satisfaction than is a perineum that has been incised and reconstructed.

Why then, is there such an emotional attachment among professionals to routine episiotomy? A prominent European professor of obstetrics and gynecology recently made the following comment on the American penchant for routine episiotomy, "Since all the physician can really do to affect the course of childbirth for the 95% of ...

mothers who are capable of giving birth without complication is to offer the mother pharmacological relief from discomfort or pain and to perform an episiotomy, there is probably an unconscious tendency for many professionals to see these practices as indispensable. "

English medical statistician, Dr. Iain Chalmers, found no significant reduction in the incidence of perineal lacerations among mothers who received routine episiotomies at birth. It would appear callous indeed for a physician or nurse-midwife to perform an episiotomy without first making an effort to avoid the need for an episiotomy by removing the mother's legs from the stirrups and bringing her up into a semi-sitting position in order to relieve tension on her perineum and enable her to push more effectively.

❏ Early Clamping or "Milking" of the Umbilical Cord

Several years ago De Marsh stated that the placental blood normally belongs to the infant and his failure to get this blood is equivalent to submitting him to a rather severe hemorrhage. Despite the fact that placental transfusion normally occurs in every corner of the world without adverse consequences there is still a great effort in the United States and Canada to deprecate the practice. One must read the literature carefully to find that placental transfusion has not been demonstrated to increase the incidence of morbidity or mortality in the placentally transfused infant.[96]
Routine early clamping or milking of the umbilical cord may appear to save the professional a few minutes time in the delivery room but neither practice has been demonstrated to be in the best interest of either the essentially un medicated mother or her infant.[76]

Placental transfusion resulting from late clamping, whereby the infant receives approximately an additional 25% of his total blood supply, is part of the physiological sequence of childbirth for most of the world's newborn infants in both developed and developing countries where the dorsal, squatting or semi-sitting position is preferred for birth. The lithotomy position for birth, preferred by the American obstetrician because it is more convenient for him, makes placental transfusion inconvenient since there is no end of the bed on which the obstetrician can place the wriggling infant. The practice of "milking" the cord in order to save 3 minutes time does not appear to be in the best interests of the newborn infant." ...

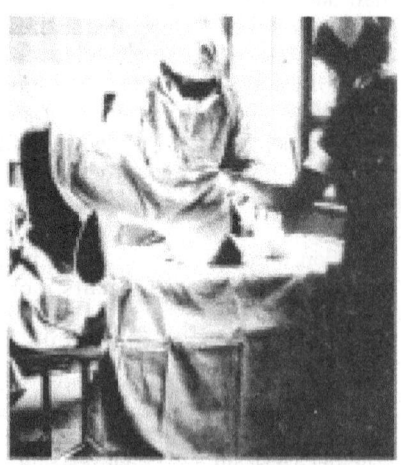

Placental transfusion occurs without added effort from the New Zealand obstetrician or midwife when the infant remains on the labor-delivery bed for about 4 minutes following birth, during which time he is given any immediate care necessary.

Early clamping has been demonstrated by research to lengthen the third stage of labor and increase the likelihood of maternal hemorrhage, retained placenta or the retention of placental fragments. [79] The latter condition frequently necessitates the mother's return to the hospital in order to stop inordinate bleeding and to prevent infection. Because early clamping tends to interfere with the spontaneous separation of the placenta, making the need for obstetrical intervention more likely, such a practice also tends to increase the incidence of fetomaternal hemorrhage or transfusion. Fetomaternal transfusion, which occurs when fetal blood cells pass into the maternal circulatory system, increases the likelihood of an Rh negative mother of an Rh positive baby developing antibodies. If a mother has already developed such antibodies fetomaternal transfusion should be avoided in order to lessen any complications for any future Rh positive fetus the mother might carry. Whether early clamping increases the incidence of anemia in the rapidly growing child has not been sufficiently investigated, but research has demonstrated that the red cell volume of late clamped full term infants increases by 47%.[96]

❑ **Routine Suctioning with a Nasogastric Tube**

Although the use of a nasogastric tube attached to a deLee trap is now a widely used method for removing mucous from the newborn infant's nasopharynx, Cordero and Hon suggest that blind suctioning with a nasogastric tube is a hazardous procedure. They point out that the procedure can cause severe cardiac arrhythmias and apnea - conditions which do not tend to develop when the suctioning is accomplished by the use of a bulb syringe.[11]

❑ **Apgar Scoring by the Accoucheur**

No one can be completely impartial in judging his own skills, no matter how objective he or she may try to be. As one pediatrician put it, "Asking the person who delivers the infant to determine that infant's score on the Apgar scale is like asking a student to fill out his own report card." In countries where obstetrical medication is the exception rather than the rule the Apgar score of the majority of newborn infants seldom falls below nine. Therefore, it would appear that an infant's Apgar score is possibly more influenced by the management of labor and delivery than the physical condition of the mother.

Although there is a "maximum dosage" level and time interval recommended by the manufacturer of most obstetrical medications there are no recommendations, guidelines or restrictions on the use of several medications administered to the mother at the same time. Nor is there any recommendation or guideline for determining safe time intervals between administration of multiple medication. ...

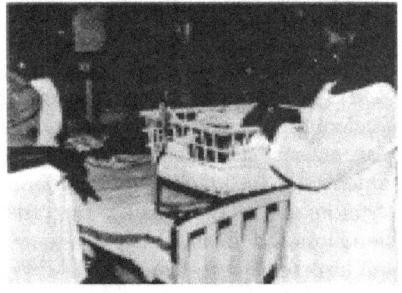

This Kenyan mother takes great pride in caring for her 18 hour old infant. She will be taught baby care, nutrition and family health during her hospital stay

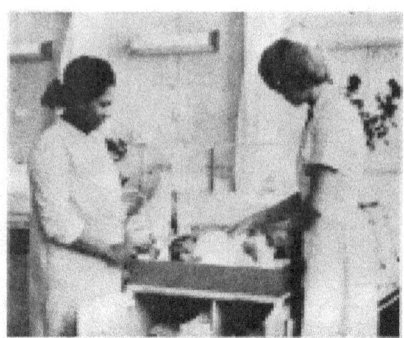

Indonesian mother receives instruction in baby care at University of Amsterdam Hospital.

A review by the hospital joint obstetric-pediatric committee of any Apgar score of 7 or below would very likely tend to improve infant outcome.

Treatment of a slow learner or retarded child may be facilitated by knowing the Apgar score of the child under observation. Since the Apgar score of an individual is not always accessible several years after birth (many hospitals discard birth records after 7 to 10 years) parents should be given a copy of their baby's Apgar score for retention, even if the score is coded.

❑ Obstetrical Intervention in Placental Expulsion

The most common mismanagement of the third stage of labor involves an attempt to hasten it.[4] Cord traction, the use of uterine stimulants such as oxytocin, ergonovene etc., manipulation of the fundus and manual removal as means of accelerating the expulsion of a reluctant placenta, are pathological procedures which tend to increase the incidence of fetomaternal transfusion, maternal blood loss and the incidence of retained afterbirth or placental fragments.[61, 78, 79, 82, 83] Such obstetrical intervention is rarely found necessary when (a) the mother has received little or no medication, (b) she has been supported to a semi-sitting position for birth and (c) where placental transfusion has reduced the volume of the placenta.[78,79]

❑ Separating the Mother from Her Newborn Infant

There is no evidence that the full term infant of a relatively unmedicated mother will suffer an abnormal drop in temperature if he is placed in his mother's arms during the recovery period.[102] Experience at Yale New Haven Hospital in Connecticut indicates that when the above procedure is followed and the mother is allowed to hold her baby for two hours or so, the infant's body temperature remains stable. In light of the present concern over the possible hazard of infant warming devices in the delivery room, perhaps we should recommend one of the most logical of warming devices - the mother's arms.

A Mother-Baby Recovery Room, staffed with skilled nursing personnel makes it possible for even the high-risk or postoperative mother to be with her baby during the first hours of life.

Recent research by Klaus [84] and Salk [85] has demonstrated that the conventional hospital postpartum routine tends to inhibit rather than engender maternal response and nurturing. The first 24 hours following birth appear to be a critical period for the establishment of the normal mother-infant bonds. Separating the mother from her infant during this time tends to interfere with the mother's normal responses to her baby. Salk suggests that the mother's increased sensitivity to her newborn ...

infant during the first 24 hours following birth may be a biochemical mechanism which is not yet understood. Both Salk and Klaus have demonstrated that maternal response and nurturing are adversely affected a full one month after birth when the mother and her baby have been restricted to the usual hospital postpartum schedule (a glimpse of the baby shortly after birth, brief contact and identification at 6 to 12 hours, and then 20 to 30 minutes every four hours for feeding). How long this initial restrictive pattern of contact adversely affects maternal behavior is yet to be assessed.

As I visit hospitals throughout the world I am always impressed by the effort made in most countries to keep mothers and their babies together from the very moment of birth. Even when there are abnormal conditions which require adjustments to be made there is still great emphasis placed on the importance of mother-baby contact during the immediate postpartum period.

❏ **Delaying the First Breast-Feeding**

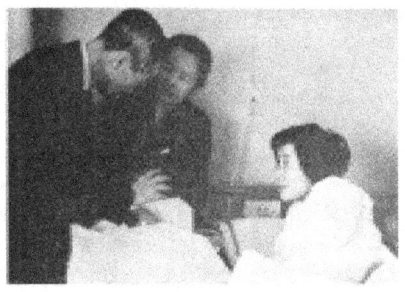

Both mother and grandmother are counseled in baby care by this Japanese physician.

The common American practice of routinely delaying the time of the first breast feeding has not been shown to be in the best interest of either the conscious mother or her newborn infant. Clinical experience with the early feeding of newborn infants has shown this practice to be safe.[86] If the mother feels well enough and the infant is capable of suckling while they are still in the delivery room then it would seem more cautious, in the event of tracheoesophogeal abnormality, to permit the infant to suckle for the first time under the watchful eye of the physician or nurse-midwife rather than delay the feeding for several hours when the expertise of the professional may not be immediately available.

In light of the many protective antibodies contained in colostrum it would seem likely that the earlier the infant's intake of species specific colostrum the sooner the antibodies can be accrued by the infant.

Research on several species of animals suggest that the earlier the newborn's intake of colostrum and maternal milk the earlier gut closure will occur. Gut closure, whereby the colostrum acts as a sealant to the intestinal lining, appears to ...

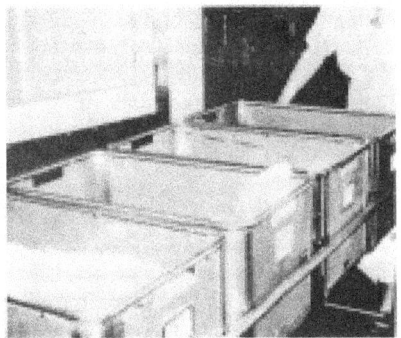

The low incidence of infection among Swedish infants appears not to be jeopardized by moving the infants to and from the nursery in this multiple infant cart.

prevent or lessen the passage of harmful bacteria or foreign protein through the intestinal lining.[87] Although similar research has not been carried out on the human infant it is not unlikely that such a similar protective mechanism exists.

❏ **Offering Water and Formula to the Breast Fed Newborn Infant**

The common American practice of giving water or formula to a newborn infant prior to the first breast-feeding or as a supplement during the first days of life has not been shown to be in the best interests of the infant. There are now indications that these practices may, in fact, be harmful. Glucose water, once the standby in every American hospital, has now been designated a potential hazard if aspirated by the newborn infant, yet it is still used in many American hospitals.

It is a comment on the American penchant for the artificial that there has never been any research carried out in the U.S. which attempts to evaluate the safety of colostrum as the infant's first intake of fluid, yet nature obviously intended the initial fluid intake of the newborn infant to be of the same consistency as the relatively thick, viscous colostrum.

Whether the human infant experiences such a gut closure, as is seen in animals, and whether the administering of water or formula initially to the infant who is to be breast-fed will interfere with normal gut closure has not been scientifically investigated. Experts in the raising of cows make great effort to see that species specific bovine colostrum, not milk or water, is the first fluid received by the newborn calf. It is ironic that we do not give the same consideration to human newborns.

Unless the physician or the nurse can be absolutely sure that an infant has no familial history of allergy it would be cautious to obtain the mother's permission before offering her infant formula in the nursery. Offering the infant formula in the nursery interferes with the normal progress of lactation in so many ways that the subject cannot be adequately discussed herein.[88] For those who wish more information on the subject I suggest you read references 57 and 89.

❏ **Restricting Newborn Infants to a Four Hour Feeding Schedule and Withholding Night Time Feedings**

Although widely spaced infant feedings may be more convenient for hospital personnel the practice of feeding a newborn infant only every four hours and not permitting the infant to breast-feed at all during the night cannot be justified on any scientific grounds. Such a regimen restricts the suckling stimulation necessary to bring about the normally rapid onset and adequate production of the mother's milk. In countries where custom permits the infant to suckle ...

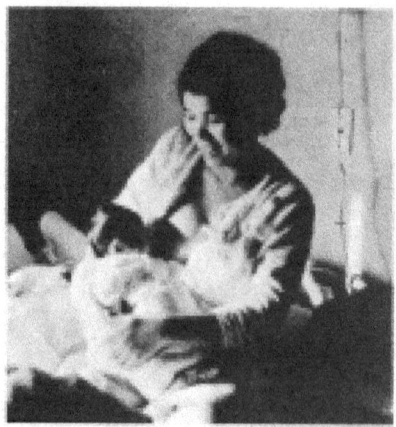

Japanese mothers are encouraged to breast-feed their baby on demand during their hospital stay.

immediately after birth and on demand from that time, first time mothers frequently begin to produce breast milk for their babies within 24 hours after birth. In contrast, in countries where hospital routines prevent normal, demand feeding from birth, mothers frequently do not produce breast milk for their babies until the third day following birth.

Widely spaced feedings, which limit the normal suckling stimulation of the breast:

1. restrict the infant's normal intake of colostrum at a time when he is most in need of the protective antibodies in colostrum,
2. increase the likelihood of dehydration in the infant by suppressing both the onset and production of breast milk
3. interfere with the maintaining of the normal, relatively constant level of glucose in the infant's blood which occurs when an infant is fed on demand
4. increase the likelihood of overdistention of the breast by interfering with the normal clearing of colostrum from the lactiferous ducts before the onset of milk,
5. increase the likelihood of poor "let down" of breast milk due to the mother's discomfort or pain resulting when the overly hungry infant tugs anxiously at his mother's engorged, unyielding breast which is over-distended with accumulated milk.

Overdistention of the breast or engorgement is a hospital acquired condition which does not occur to any comparable degree in cultures where mothers are permitted to breast-feed their babies on demand from birth.[90]

Physiological jaundice, which, if it does occur, usually appears about the third day of life, appears to be quite common among infants in those cultures where breast-feeding predominates. The switching of an infant from his mother's milk to foreign protein because he shows evidence of physiological jaundice is a practice which has not been justified by scientific research.[91]

A scientific evaluation of the relationship of prenatal diuretics and other pharmacologic agents to the incidence of postnatal jaundice should be carried out.

❏ Preventing Early Father-Child Contact

Permitting fathers to hold their newborn infants immediately following birth and during the postpartum hospital stay has not been shown by research or clinical experience to increase the incidence of infection among newborns, even when those infants are returned to a regular or central nursery. Yet, only in the eastern European countries is the father permitted less involvement in the immediate postpartum period than in the United States (eastern European fathers are usually not permitted to enter beyond the foyer of the maternity hospital and are not allowed to see their wives or ...

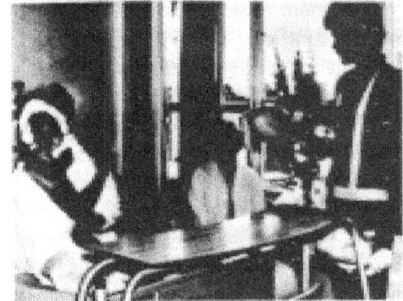

Like most children in the rest of the world, this New Zealand toddler is permitted to be with her mother and new sibling during the postpartum hospital stay in order to minimize the trauma of separation for the toddler.

babies for the entire 7 to 9 day stay). Research has consistently confirmed the fact that the greatest sources of infection to the newborn infant are the nursery and nursery personnel.[92,93] One has only to observe a mother holding her newborn infant against her bathrobe, which has probably been exposed to abundant hospital borne bacteria, to realize the fallacy of preventing a father from holding his baby during the hospital stay.

❏ **Assigning Nursing Personnel to Mothers or to Babies (rather than to mother-baby couples)**

The traditional American system of assigning postpartum nurses to mothers and nursery nurses to babies has done much to distort the normal pattern of initial mother-baby interaction.[85] The European concept of assigning nursing personnel to care for mother-baby couples, then letting them care for their assigned babies in the mothers' rooms or in the nursery, has not been shown to increase the incidence of infection. The latter pattern of assignment has been approved by the Committee on Fetus and Newborn of the American Academy of Pediatrics.[22]

❏ **Restricting Intermittent Rooming-In to Specific Room Requirements**

Throughout the world great effort is made to keep mothers and babies together in the hospital, no matter how inconvenient the accommodations. There is no research or evidence which indicates that intermittent rooming-in should be restricted to private rooms or to rooms which have a sink, or which provide at least 80 square feet for mother and baby. Such requirements are based on conjecture and not controlled evaluation. Nor is there any scientific support for requiring that each room used for intermittent rooming-in

be supplied with a covered diaper receptacle. A simple system, whereby soiled diapers and baby linen are placed in plastic bags which are tied to the crib (for the mother's convenience) and then changed at the end of each shift has been found to be safe. This system would appear less likely to be a source of infection than using communal diaper receptacles and is far less expensive for the hospital.

❏ **Restricting Sibling Visitation**

The common American practice of prohibiting toddlers and children from visiting their mothers during the hospital stay is an emotional hardship on both the mothers and their children and is unsupported by scientific research or evidence. Experience in other countries and in several hospitals here in the ...

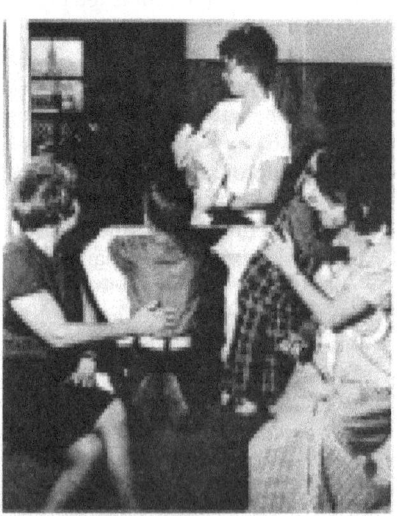

In a "Childrens' Visiting Area", cordoned off from a hallway across from an elevator, an American toddler cuddles her mother while her grandmother and older brother admire their new family member.

United States suggests that where sibling visitation is permitted a short explanation as to the importance of not bringing suspect illnesses into the hospital seems to be effective in controlling infection.

Summary

As mentioned previously, most of the practices discussed above have developed not from a lack of concern for the well being of the mother and baby but from a lack of awareness as to the problems which can arise from each progressive digression from the normal childbearing experience. Like a snowball rolling down hill, as one unphysiological practice is employed, for one reason or another, another frequently becomes necessary to counteract some of the disadvantages,
large or small, inherent in the previous procedure.

The higher incidence of fetal, neonatal and maternal deaths occurring in our large urban hospitals, as opposed to our smaller community hospitals,[94] is undoubtedly due, in part, to the greater proportion of high risk mothers in the urban areas. But we in the United States must stop looking for scapegoats and face up to the fact that by individualizing the care offered to maternity patients much can be done immediately to improve infant outcome without the slightest outlay of capital

There is currently an increasing emphasis on consolidating maternity facilities. However, we do not see the consolidation of community obstetrical facilities as being always in the best interest of the vast majority of mothers who are capable of giving birth without complications. There should, of course, be centers where those mothers who have had no prenatal care or who are anticipated to be obstetrical risks can be properly cared for. But to insist that every healthy mother must go to a major maternity facility which is unnecessary for her needs and inconvenient for her family, and where she is very apt to be "lost in the crowd," will only spur the growing trend in the United States toward professionally unattended home births.

Throughout the United States the current inclination of many expectant parents is to seek out, to "shop around" for the type of physician and hospital they feel they need in order to have the type of childbearing experience they want. They not only want a doctor who will support them in their efforts to have a prepared, natural birth, with a minimum of or no medication, they also want a hospital which offers education for childbearing and a supportive family-centered atmosphere. These expectant mothers appreciate the availability of such facilities as an Early Labor Lounge, a dual purpose Labor-Delivery Room, a Mother-Baby Recovery Room, and a Children's Visiting Room if they have older children. But most of all they want a supportive atmosphere in which they can share the childbearing experience to the extent that they desire and one which makes an effort to meet the individual needs of the mother, the father and their newborn baby as they form their family bonds during the hospital stay.

By working together in an interdisciplinary effort the professional and lay members of the American Academy of Husband-Coached Childbirth, National Childbirth Trust of Great Britain and The Parents' Centers of both New Zealand and Australia, have served as catalysts to the improvement of maternity care throughout much of the world. We stand united in the belief that parents should be educated and prepared for childbearing ...

and then be given the freedom to participate effectively in the birth of their children in order to insure the quality of life's beginning.

1976 Postscript

During the spring of 1974 and 1975 two major medical conferences were held which dealt with the issues of birth trauma and birth injury and their effect on the development of the child. The conferences, entitled Part I and Part II of "OBSTETRICAL MANAGEMENT and INFANT OUTCOME: Implications for Future Mental and Physical Development" were sponsored by the American Foundation for Maternal and Child Health, 30 Beekman Place, New York N.Y. The proceedings of these conferences, which will be published late in 1976, underscore the hazards of the routine use of obstetrical medication, the elective induction and chemical stimulation of labor and the artificial rupture of embranes. These *(continued on page 32)*

References

1. Chase, H.: "Ranking Countries by Infant Mortality Rates," Public Health Reports, 84:19-27, 1969.
2. Wegman, M.: "Annual Summary of Vital Statistics - 1969," Pediatrics, 47:461-464, 1971.
3. Debdas. A. and Chowdhury, R.: "Fetal Distress and pH Value of Umbilical Cord Blood," Amer. J. Obstet. & Gynec., 107:1044, 1970.
4. Hellman, L. & Pritchard, J.: *Williams Obstetrics*, 14th Ed. Appleton, Century-Crofts, New York, 1971.
5. McCance, R.: "The Maintenance of Stability in the Newborn," Arch. Dis. Childh.., 34:361-370, 1959
6. Bowes, W. et al: "The Effects of Obstetrical Medication on Fetus and Infant," Monographs of the Society for Research in Child Development, No. 137, Vol. 35, June 1970.
7. Levy, B., Wilkinson, F. and Marine, W.: "Reducing Neonatal Mortality Rate with Nurse Midwives," Am. J. Obstet. Gynec., 109:50-58, 1971.
8. Windle, W.: "Brain Damage by Asphyxia at Birth," Scient. Amer. 17-83, Oct. 1969.
9. Brazelton, T.B.,: "Effect of Maternal Medication on the Neonate and his Behavior," J. Pediat., 58:513-518, 1961.
10. Kron, R.: "Newborn Sucking Behavior Affected by Obstetric Sedation," Pediatrics, 37:1012-1016, 1966.
11. Adamsons, K. and Joelsson, I.: "The Effects of Pharmacological Agents Upon the Fetus and Newborn," Am. J. Obstet. & Gynec., 96:437- 460, 1966.
12. Baker, J.: "The Effects of Drugs on the Fetus," Pharm. Review, 12:37-90, 1960.
13. Flowers, C.: *Obstetric Analgesia and Anesthesia*, Hoeber, Harper & Row, N.Y., 1967.
14. Grimwade, J. et al.: "Human Fetal Heart Rate Change and Movement in Response to Sound and Vibration," Am. J. Obltet. cl Gynec., 109:86-90, 1971.
15. James, L.S.: "The Effects of Pain Relief for Labor and Delivery on the Fetus and Newborn," Anesthesiology, 21 :405-430, 1960.
16. Lewis, M. et al: "Individual Differences in Attention," Amer. J. Dis. Child., 113:461-465, 1967.
17. Ploman, L. and Penson, B.: "On the Transfer of Barbiturates to the Human Fetus and their Accumulation in Some of its Vital Organs," J. Obstet. Gynaec., Brit. Emp., 64:706- 711, 1967.
18. Vasicky, A.: "Fetal Bradycardia after Paracervical Block," Obstet. Gynec. 38:500- 512n 1971.
19. Roaefsky, J. and Peteniel, M.: "Perinatal Deaths Associated with. Mepivacaine Paracervical Block Anesthesia in Labor," N.E.J. Med., 278:530-533, 1968.
20. Werboff, J. and Kelner, R.: *Learning Deficits of Offspring after Administration of Tranquilllizing Drugs to the Mothers*," Nature 197:106-107, 1963.
21. Sinclair, J. et al.: "Intoxication of the Fetus by a Local Anesthetic," N.E.J. of Med. 273:1173- 1177, 1965.
22. Haire, D. Haire, J.: *Implementing Family Centered Maternity Care with a Central Nursery*, Publ, Internnational Childbirth Ed. Assn., Milwaukee. Wisconsin, 1971.
23. Richards, M. and Bernal, J.: "Effects of Obstetric Medication on Mother-Infant Interaction and Infant Development," III International Congress of Psycho. Med. in Obstet. and Gynec., London, April 1971.
24. Johnson, W.: "Regionals can Prolong Labor," Medical World New .. Oct. 15, 1971.
25. Potter, N. cl MacDonald, R.: "Obstetric Consequences of Epidural Analgesia in Nulliparous Patients," Lancet, I: 1031-1 034, May 22, 1971.
26. Gordon, H.: "Fetal Bradycardia after Paracervical Block," N.EJ. of Med., 97:910- 914, 1968.
27. Rosefsky, J. and Petersiel, M.: "Perinatal Deaths Associated with Mepivacaine Paracervical Block Anethesia · in Labor," N.E.J. Med .. 278:530- 533, 1968.
28. Towbin, A: "Spinal Cord and Brain Stem Injuries at Birth," Arch. Path. 77:620~32, 1964.

29. Hubinont, P. et al: *"Effects of Vacuum Extractor and Obstetrical Forceps on the Fetus and Newborn - A Comparison,"* V World Congress Gynaec. & Obstet., Sydney, Australia, 1967.
30. Hon, E.: *"Direct Monitoring of the Fetal Heart,"* Hosp. Prac. 91-97, Sept. 1970.
31. Hon, E. and Quilligan, E.: *"Electronic Evaluation of Fetal Heart Rate,"* Clin. Obst. & Gynec. 145-167, March, 1968.
32. MacKenzie, L.: *"Malpractice Hazards in Obstetrics and Gynecology,"* N.Y. State J. of Med. 1877-1879, August I, 1971.
33. Glaser, J.: *"The Dietary Prophylaxis of Allergic Diseases in Infancy,"* J. Asthma Research, 3:199-208, 1966.
34. Rose, A.H. and Rose, A., Jr.: *Bronchial Asthma: Its Diagnosis and Treatment*, Charles C. Thomas Pub., Springfield, IL., 1963.
35. Baum, J.: *"Nutritional Value of Human Milk,"* Obstet. & Gynec., 37:126-130, 1971.
36. Jelliffe, D. & Jelliffe E.: *"The Uniqueness of Human Milk: An Overview,"* Amer. J. Clin. Nutr., 24:1013-1024, August, 1971.
37. Robinson, M.: *"Infant Morbidity and Mortality: A Study of 3266 Infants,"* Lancet. 260:788.
38. Hodes, H.: *"Colostrum: A Valuable Source of Antibodies,"* Ob-Gyn. Observer, 3:7, 1964.
39. Michaels, R.: *"Studies of Antiviral Factors in Human Milk and Serum,"* J. Immunology, 94:262-263, 1965.
40. Svirsky-Gross, St.: *"Pathogenic Strains of Coli (0, 111) Among Prematures and The Use of Human Milk in Controlling the Outbreak of Diarrhea,"* Ann. Paediat., 190:109-115, 1958.
41. Kenny, J. et al: *"Bacterial and 'Viral Coproantibodies in Breast-Fed Infants,"* Pediatrics, 39:202-213, 1967.
42. Anderson, D. and Mike, E.: *"Diet Therapy in the Celiac Syndrome,"* J. Amer. Dietetic Assn. 31:340-346, 1955.
43. DiSant'Agnese" P. and Jones, W.: *"The Celiac Syndrome (Malabsorption) in Pediatrics,"* J.A.M.A., 180:308-316, 1962.
44. Frogatt, P. et al: *"Epidemiology of Sudden Unexpected Death in Infants (Cot Death) in Northern Ireland,"* Brit. J. Prevo Soc. Med: 25:119-134, 1971.
45. Bergman, A. et al: *Sudden Infant Death Syndrome*, Proc. 2nd Int'\. Conf. Sudden Death in Infants, PUb. Un. Washington Press, Seattle, 1970.
46. Widdowson, E. et a\.: *"Absorption, Excretion, and Retention of Strontium by Breast-Fed and Bottle-Fed Babies,"* Lancet, 941-944, Oct. 1960.
47. Straub, C. and Murthy, G.: *"A Comparison of Sr 90 Component of Human and Cow's Milk,"* Pediatrics, 36:732-735, 1965.
48. Tank, G.: *"Relation of Diet to Variation of Dental Caries,"* J. Amer. Dental Ass'n, 70:394-403, 1965.
49. Graber, T.: *"Malocclusion: Extrinsic or General Factors"* in Orthodontics: Principles and Practice, Saunders Co., Philadelphia, 1962.
50. Marks, M.: *"Allergy in Relation to Orofacial Dental Deformities in Children,"* J. Allergy, 36:293-302, 1965.
51. Osborn, G.R.: *"Stages in Development of Coronary Disease Observed from 1500 Young Subjects: Relation of Hypotension and Infant Feeding to Aeriology,"* Le Role De La Paroi Arterielle Dans L'Atherogeneses, Editions due Centre National de la Recherche Scientific, 169:93-139, Paris, 1968.
52. Foman, S.: *"A Pediatrician Looks at Early Nutrition,"* Bull. N.Y. Acad. Med., 47:569-578, 1971.
53. Acheson, E. and Truelove, S.: *"Early Weaning in the Aetiology of Ulcerative Colitis,"* Brit. Med. J., 929-933, Oct., 1961.
54. Sturman, J. et al: *"Absence of Cystathionase in Human Fetal Liver: Is Cystine Essential?,"* Science, 169:74-75, 1970.
55. Crosse, V. et al.; *"The Value of Human Milk Compared with other Feeds for Premature Infants,"* Arch. Dis. Childh., 29:178-195,1954.
56. Paffenbarger, Jr., R.: *"Susceptibility to Late Postpartum Hemorrhage,"* Am. J. Obstet. & Gynec., 87:263-267, 1963.
57. Haire, D. & Haire, J.: *"The Nurse's Contribution to Successful Breast-Feeding,"* Int'l Childbirth Ed. Ass'n, Milwaukee, Wisconsin, 1971.
58. Enkin, M. et al: *"An Adequately Controlled Study of the Effectiveness of P.P.M. Training,"* III Int'I Congress of Psycho. Med. in Obstet. & Gynec., London, April, 1971.
59. Fields, H.: *"Complications of Elective Induction,"* Obstet. & Gyneco., 15:476-480, 1960.
60. Fields, H.: *"Induction of Labor: Methods, Hazards, Complications and Contraindications,"* Hospital Topics, 63-68, Dec. 1968.
61. Beer, A.: *"Fetal Erythrocytes in Maternal Circulation of 155 Rh-Negative Women,"* Obstet. & Gynec., 34:143-150, 1969.
62. Butler, N.: *"A National Long Term Study of Perinatal Hazards,"* Sixth World Congress, Fed. Int. Gynec. & Obstet., 1970.
63. Kelly, J.: *"Effect of Fear Upon Uterine Motility,"* Am. J. Obstet. Gynec., 83:576-581, 1962.
64. Veland, K. & Hansen, J.: *"Maternal Cardiovascular Dynamics,* Posture & Uterine Contractions," AM. J. Obstet. & Gynec., 103:1, Jan. 1969.
65. Burchell, R.: *"Predelivery Removal of Pubic Hair,"* Obstet. & Gynec., 24:272-273, 1964.
66. Kantor, H., et al: *"Value of Shaving the Pudendal-Perineal Area in Delivery Preparation,"* Obstet. & Gynec., 25:509-512, 1965.
67. American Academy of Pediatrics, *Standards and*

Recommendations for Hospital Care of Newborn Infants, Fifth Edition, 1971.
68. Blankfield, A.: "The Optimum Position for Childbirth," Med. J. Australia, 2:666-668, 1965.
69. Howard, F.H.: "Delivery in the Physiologic Position," Obstet. & Gynec., II :318-322, 1958.
70. Gritsiuk, I.: "Position in Labor," Ob-Gyn Observer, Sept. 1968.
71. Newton, N. and Newton M. "The Propped Position for the Second Stage of Labor," Obstet. & Gynec., 15:28-34, 1960.
72. Naroll, F., Naroll, R. and Howard F.: "Position of Women in Childbirth," Am. J. Obstet. & Gynec., 82:943-954, 1961.
73. Richardson, S. and Guttmacher, A. (Eds.): "Childbearing - Its Social and Psychological Aspects," Williams and Wilkins Co., Baltimore, Md., 1967.
74. Cooperman, N., Rubovits, F., and Hesser, F.: "Oxygen Saturation in the Newborn Infant," Am. J. Obstet. & Gynec., 81 :385-394, 1961.
75. Demarsh, Q., Alt, H. and Windle, W.: "The Effect of Depriving the Infant of Its Placental Blood," J.A.M.A., 116:2568-2573, 1941.
76. Avery, M.: "Decreased Blood Volume," The Lung and Its Disorders in the Newborn Infant, 1:130-131, W.B. Saunders Co., Philadelphia.
77. Duckman, S., et al: "The Importance of Gravity in Delayed Ligation of the Umbilical Cord," Am. J. Obstet. & Gynec., 66:1214-1223, 1953.
78. Walsh, S.: "Maternal Effects of Early and Late Clamping of the Umbilical Cord," Lancet, 1:996-997, 1968.
79. Botha, M.: "The Management of the Umbilical Cord in Labour," S. Afr. J. Obstet. 6(2):30-33, 1968.
80. Moss, A. and Monset-Couchard, M.: "Placental Transfusion: Early Versus Late Clamping of the Umbilical Cord," Pediatrics 40:109-126, 1967.
81. Cordero, L. and Hon, E.: "Neonatal Bradycardia Fo 110 wing Nasopharyngeal Stimulation," J. Pediat., 78:441-447, 1971.
82. Doolittle, J. & Moritz, c.: "Prevention of Erythroblastosis by an Obstetric Technic," Obstet. & Gynec., 27:529-531, 1966.
83. Weinstein, L., Farabow, W. and Gusdon, J.: "Third Stage of Labor and Transplacental Hemorrhage," Obstet. & Gynec., 37:90-93, 1971.
84. Klaus, M. et al: "Maternal Attachment Importance of the First Post-Partum Days," N.E.J. of Med. 286:460-463, March 2, 1972.
85. Salk, L.: "The Critical Nature of the Post Partum Period in the Human for the Establishment of the Mother-Infant Bond: A Controlled Study," Dis. Ner. Sys., 31 :Suppl: 110-116, Nov. 1970.
86. Eppink, H.: "Time of Initial Breast Feeding Surveyed in Michigan Hospitals," Hospital Topics, 116-117, June 1968.
87. Lecce, J. et al.: "Effect of Feeding Colostral and Milk Components on the Cessation of Intestinal Absorption of Large Molecules Closure in Neonatal Pigs," J. Nutrition, 78:263-268, 1962.
88. Newton, M. and Newton, N.: "Normal Course and Management of Lactation," Clin. Obst. and Gynec., 5:44-63, 1962.
89. Newton, M.: "Human Lactation," in Milk: The Mammary Gland and its Secretion, Vol. I, edited by S. Kon and A. Cowie, N.Y. Academic Press, 1961.
90' Newton, M. and Newton, N.: "Postpartum Engorgement of the Breast," Am. J. Obstet. and Gynec., 61 :664-667, 1951.
91. Gartner, L. and Arias, I.: 'Jaundice in Breast-Fed Neonates" J.AM.A p. 746, Nov. 1. 1971.
Pediat., 68:54-66, 1966.
92. Gezon, H., et al: "Some Controversial Aspects in the Epidemiology of Hospital Nursery Staphylococcal Infections," Amer. J. of Public Health, 50:473-484, 1960.
93. Ravenholt, R. and LaVeck, G.: "Staphylococcal Disease-An Obstetric, Pediatric & Community Problem," Amer. J. of Public Health, 46:1287-1296, 1956.
94. Bishop, E.: "The National Study of Maternity Care," Obstet. & Gynec. ;745-750, 1971.
95. White, G. Emergency Childbirth: A Manual. Pub. by Police Training Foundation, Franklin Park, Illinois.
96. Saigal, S. et al: "Placental Transfusion and Hyperbilirubinemia in the Premature." Pediatrics, 49:406-419, 1972.
97. Montagu, A: *Prenatal Influences*, C.C. Thomas, Springfield, Md, 1962.
98. Newton, N.: "The Effects of Disturbance on Labor." Amer. J. Obstet. and Gynec. 101:1096-1102, 1968.
99. Bland, R.: "Otitis Media in the First Six Weeks of Life: Diagnosis, Bacteriology and Management," Pediatrics 49:187-197, 1972.
100. Gellis, S.: "Crossing the Birth Barrier," Hosp. Practice, 1:28-31, Oct. 1966.
101. Hoff, F.: "Natural Childbirth: How Any Nurse Can Help" Am. J. Nursing, 69:1451-1453, 1969.
102. Dahm, L. and James, L.: "Newborn Temperature: Heat Loss in Delivery Room, ": Pediatrics 49:504-513, 1972.

Additional related references may be found in Reference No. 22 above. For those who do not have access to a medical library the research papers listed above may usually be obtained through your public library, either directly or by interlibrary loan. For additional references on a specific subject, consult Index Medicus at your local library.
See also *Physicians Desk Reference* for information on a specific medication.

Note: There are no states with laws which prevent a pharmacist from giving a patient a copy of the Package Insert (information sheet) which ccompanies drugs released or approved by the FDA.

1976 Postscript (continued from page 29)

conferences provided scientific and statistical data which give further support to the research described in "The Cultural Warping of Childbirth."

During the latter part of 1972 the Collaborative Perinatal Study, sponsored by the National Institute of Neurological Diseases and Stroke, issued its first major report entitled "THE WOMEN and THEIR PREGNANCIES," published by W. Saunders and Co. The Study, which followed over 50,000 infants from birth to one year of age, reported some surprising facts when they compared the incidence of significant neurologic damage in children at one year of age. The study found that there was a slightly greater incidence of neurologic damage among white children than among black children of the same age.

These findings are not so startling when one considers that, although the incidence of low birth weight, prematurity and undernutrition is decidedly greater among our black population, black patients, who are more often clinic patients, traditionally receive less medication during labor and birth. (In one New York City hospital during 1970, there was twice the incidence of depressed babies among private patients as among clinic patients.)

The Committee on Drugs of the American Academy of Pediatrics has issued a warning that there is no drug, whether over-the-counter remedy or prescription drug, which, when taken by or administered to a childbearing woman, has been proven safe for the unborn child (Pediatrics, 51:297-299, 1973). This statement led us to probe into the workings of the U.S. Food and Drug Administration (FDA) and we have been shocked to learn that, according to the Director of the Bureau of Drugs of the FDA, the criteria used by the FDA for determining the safety of drugs administered during labor and delivery have not included a requirement that long-term safety be shown for the mental and neurological development of the child.

There is no animal which duplicates human physiology, as evidenced by the Thalidomide tragedy. Therefore, tests on animals cannot be accepted as conclusive evidence of the short term and long term effects of a drug or device on the child exposed to the product in utero.

Our probe into the workings of the FDA brought out several frightening facts. The vast majority of drugs prescribed for, or administered to pregnant, parturient or lactating women were approved for marketing by the FDA prior to the 1962 amendments to the Act. Prior to these amendments a drug manufacturer merely had to register the drug with the FDA and wait for a relatively short period of time; then if there were no strong objections the drug was approved for marketing by the FDA.

Although the FDA has the authority to require a manufacturer to inform the physician or pharmacist in the package insert, which accompanies every drug covered by the Act, that the drug has not been tested for its short and long term effects on the physical, neurological and mental development of the child, the FDA has not exercised this authority for all drugs. Nor has the FDA required a long-term follow-up of children exposed to ultrasound in utero.

The present FDA regulations allow massive unmonitored experimentation with human lives and mental potential. Rather than requiring a manufacturer to test his product on a limited number of subjects who are fully aware that the long term effects of the product under investigation are unknown, the FDA is allowing the uninformed general public to establish the long-term safety or hazards of a given product. Millions of American children have been allowed to be exposed to drugs in utero without scientifically valid sequential evaluations being carried out on the child so exposed. Unfortunately the reporting of an adverse drug reaction by a physician to the FDA is strictly voluntary.

It has become increasingly evident that the so-called "judicious use" of obstetric drugs can only be determined after the child is born, when it may be too late to correct an error in judgment. The fallacy of judging the safety of a drug or procedure only by its short term effects has been made tragically evident by the fact that the drug diethylstilbestrol, given to more than 1,000,000 pregnant American women in order to forestall premature labor, has now been linked statistically to a significantly increased incidence of cancer of the reproductive system in female offspring 10 to 20 years after exposure to the drug in utero. The effect of the drug on male offspring is only now becoming evident.

We cannot look to the Collaborative Perinatal Study to guide us to a safe form of analgesic or anesthetic agent for childbearing, for the Collaborative Study did not include a sufficient control group of normal, un-medicated mothers and their babies which could have served as a base line against which to measure deviations in normal newborn behavior and response.

We have good reason to look at every aspect of care that may affect the future potential of the human intellect since - One in every 35 children born in the United States today will eventually be diagnosed as retarded. In addition, one in every 10 to 17 children in the United States is afflicted by some form of brain dysfunction or learning disability.

While we are told of the value of eliminating small and medium sized obstetric services we find that a national survey of U.S. obstetric services carried out by the American College of Obstetricians and Gynecologists reveals that, in general, the larger the obstetric service the greater the rate of infant and maternal deaths, and that the stronger the affiliation between the obstetric service and a medical school the greater the rate of infant and maternal deaths. Undoubtedly some of these deaths result from the fact that there is a greater incidence of high-risk mothers in larger, teaching hospitals, but it is also possible that the greater tendency to intervene in the normal progress of labor and birth in these institutions in order to provide teaching opportunities contributes to these statistics and may also result in a disproportionately high incidence of neurologically damaged children.

Improving the Outcome of Pregnancy Through Science

Statement by Doris Haire, President
American Foundation for Maternal and Child Health, New York
to the FDA Science Board
November 17, 2000

I appreciate this opportunity to share my concerns with the members of the FDA Science Board, and to ask the Board to urge the FDA to create an Interdisciplinary Obstetric Advisory Board comprised of pediatricians, pediatric neurologists, behavioral scientists, midwives, obstetric nurses and obstetricians to evaluate the safety of drugs to be administered to pregnant and parturient women. The FDA can not expect a Maternal Health Drug Advisory Committee made up almost exclusively of obstetricians to be objective about the drugs they have administered to their patients. Such a group does not have the training or expertise to determine the delayed effects of the drugs they administer to parturients on the long-term neurologic development of the exposed offspring. I have heard obstetricians in that committee remind the group that there could be "serious repercussions" for obstetricians if the committee were to recommend that a drug previously approved by that committee be removed from the market.

The fact that the makers of Pitocin, Marcaine, Sublimaze and other drugs commonly used in obstetric care have chosen to remove their labels from the Physicians Desk Reference only adds to our conviction that they wish to withhold ready information regarding the risks of their drugs, not only from the public, but the doctors and other health care providers themselves. Most nurses and midwives who are asked to administer these drugs are refused when they ask the hospital pharmacy for a copy of the package inserts.

I am concerned that as the number of children with learning disability, autism, dyslexia, attention deficit, and hyperactivity continue to mount to a frightening number, the FDA does not appear to be making a strong endeavor to see if obstetric related drugs contribute to these problems. For some reason scientists seem to have let the science of human parturition slip through the cracks. As evidence of this scientific vacuum, a recent *Report of the Task Force on the NIH Women's Health Research Agenda for the 21st Century* failed to mention the need to improve the safety of childbirth for the woman and her baby and the need to determine the potential adverse effects of obstetric drugs and interventions on the neurologic development of the exposed offspring.

In light of the soaring rate of autistic children (500% increase in some states) and otherwise neurologically impaired children during the last ten years, it behooves the FDA to question whether cervical ripeners, uterine stimulants and ...

the various pain relieving drugs administered to the parturient permanently alter the brain chemistry of the fetus and newborn sufficiently to
interfere with the normal dendritic arborization within the infant's brain. Virtually all of the drugs administered to the parturient cross the placenta, enter the circulatory system and brain of the fetus and newborn infant where the drugs or their metabolites remain for days, if not weeks.

It is ironic that women who do not wish to become pregnant are provided a package insert with their contraceptive drugs to insure that they understand the risks of taking the drug. Yet the woman who wishes to have a safe birth experience for her baby, as well as herself, receives no package insert advising her of the known or potential risks to her and her baby.

I urge the FDA Science Board to recommend that the FDA require that package inserts be made a available on request to all expectant mothers who wish to know about the drugs they will be offered during pregnancy, labor, delivery, and postpartum.

OXYTOCIN: Consider the information the doctor receives regarding the risks of oxytocin. The manufacturer of oxytocin warns the provider in the
package insert:
"Maternal deaths due to hypertensive episodes, subarachnoid hemorrhage, rupture of the uterus, fetal deaths and permanent CNS or brain damage of the infant due to various causes have been reported to be associated with the use of parenteral oxytocic drugs for induction of labor or for augmentation in the first and second stages of labor."

In addition to the more benign effects of uterine stimulants, such as nausea and vomiting, the American manufacturer of Pitocin (oxytocin) points out in its package insert that oxytocin can cause:
 (a) maternal hypertensive episodes
 (b) subarachnoid hemorrhage
 (c) anaphylactic reaction
 (d) postpartum hemorrhage
 (e) cardiac arrhythmias
 (f) fatal afibrinogenemia
 (g) premature ventricular contraction
 (h) pelvic hematoma
 (i) uterine hypertonicity
 (j) uterine spasm
 (k) tetanic contractions
 (l) uterine rupture

(m) increased blood loss
(n) convulsions
(o) coma
(p) fatal oxytocin-induced water intoxication

The following adverse effects of maternally administered oxytocin have been reported in the fetus or infant:
(a) bradycardia
(b) premature ventricular contractions and other arrhythmias
(c) low 5 minute Apgar scores
(d) neonatal jaundice
(e) neonatal retinal hemorrhage
(f) permanent central nervous system or brain damage
(d) fetal death

Uterine stimulants which foreshorten the oxygen-replenishing intervals between contractions, by making the contractions too long, too strong, or too close together, increase the likelihood that fetal brain cells will die. The situation is somewhat analogous to holding an infant under the surface of the water, allowing the infant to come to the surface to gasp for air, but not to breathe. All of these effects increase the possibility of neurologic insult to the fetus. No one really knows how often these adverse effects occur because there is no law or regulation in any country which requires the doctor to report an adverse drug reaction to the country's drug regulating agency, even if the patient dies. I was pleased to note that this flaw in our system made the front page of yesterday's Los Angeles Times.

There are now growing indications that oxytocin may contribute to the incidence of autism. But is it the oxytocin or is it the drug used in epidurals that then precipitates the need for oxytocin.?

EPIDURAL ANESTHESIA

Consider the following information which the U.S. Food and Drug Administration currently requires the manufacturer of bupivacaine hcl (Marcaine) to provide those care givers licensed to administer epidural anesthesia. The government approved labeling for bupivacaine hcl (Marcaine) reads:

LABOR AND DELIVERY:

Local anesthetics rapidly cross the placenta, and when used for epidural, caudal or pudendal block anesthesia, can cause varying degrees of maternal, fetal and neonatal toxicity... Adverse reactions in the parturient, fetus and neonate involve alteration of the central nervous system, peripheral vascular tone and cardiac function..." Under "**ADVERSE REACTIONS. Neurologic**" the official labeling continues:

> "Neurologic effects following epidural or caudal anesthesia may include spinal block of varying magnitude (including high or total spinal block); hypotension secondary to spinal block; urinary retention; fecal and urinary incontinence; loss of perineal sensation and sexual function; persistent anesthesia; paresthesia, weakness, paralysis of the lower extremities and loss of sphincter control all of which may have slow, incomplete or no recovery; headache; backache; septic meningitis; meningismus; slowing of labor; in-creased incidence of forceps delivery; and cranial nerve palsies due to traction on nerves from loss of cerebrospinal fluid.....Neurologic effects fol-lowing other procedures or routes of administration may include persistent anesthesia, paresthesia, weakness, paralysis, all of which may have slow, incomplete, or no recovery."

EPIDURAL ANESTHESIA AND CESAREAN SECTION

A randomized controlled prospective trial carried out by Thorp and colleagues has shown a ten fold increase in the rate of cesarean section among mothers who received a labor epidural. Separate investigations by Newton and others have shown that epidural analgesia can cause disruptions in normal uterine function that cannot be completely corrected by the use of oxytocin and can double the rate of stress incontinence.

Drug manufacturers would have you believe that the incidence and degree of toxicity of a drug depends only upon the procedure performed, the type and amount of drug used, and the technique of drug administration. What they fail to tell the provider is that gestational age, condition of the fetus, previous and concomitant exposure to other drugs, relative hypoxia and various pathological conditions can affect how a drug given to the mother will affect her fetus during labor, birth and the infant's development following birth. Hypoxemia and a resulting build up of lactic acid in the fetal blood during labor and birth can in-crease the uptake of a maternal drug by the fetal brain and heart.

EFFECT OF EPIDURAL ANESTHESIA ON NEWBORN

Rosenblatt and her fellow investigators found that bupivacaine administered to the mother during labor can have prolonged adverse effects on the subsequent development of the exposed offspring. The investigators found that newborn infants with greater exposure to bupivacaine in utero were more likely to be cyanotic and unresponsive. They also found that visual skills and alertness decreased significantly with increases in the cord blood concentration of bupivacaine, particularly on the first day of life, but also throughout the next six weeks. Adverse effects of bupivacaine levels on the infant's motor organization, his ability to control his own state of consciousness and his physiological response to stress were also observed. In 1992 Sepkoski and colleagues carried out a similar investigation which supports the earlier findings of Rosenblatt et al.

These findings underscore the importance of managing the woman's labor in a way that will avoid the need for pitocin and the pain relieving drugs that are often administered to help the women cope with the chemically intensified contractions.

As early as 1975 the FDA acknowledged in its "General Considerations for the Clinical Evaluation of Drugs in Infants and Children" that drugs trapped in the infant's brain at birth have the potential to adversely affect the rapidly developing nerve circuitry of the brain and central nervous system by altering:
a) the rate at which the nerve cells in the brain mature,
b) the process by which the brain cells develop individual characteristic and capacity to carry out specific functions,
c) the process by which the brain cells are guided into their proper place within the brain and central nervous system,
d) the interconnection of the branch-like nerve fibers as the circuitry of the brain is formed, and
e) the forming of the insulating sheath of myelin (fat-like) substance around the nerve fibers which help to assure that the nerve impulses - the message to and from the brain - will travel their normal routes at the normal rate of speed.

Now the work of Zheng, Heintz, and Hatten reaffirms that the migration of neurons along the glial fibers within the brain can be altered by changing the normal chemistry of the rapidly developing brain.

At no other time in an individual's life is his or her brain more vulnerable to alteration, trauma, and permanent injury than during the hours which surround that individual's birth. The nerve circuity of the brain and central nervous system of the fetus is rapidly developing as labor begins, making these complex structures vulnerable to permanent alteration or damage from the drugs and procedures administered to the mother during that time.

If the FDA is to be truly responsible to the citizens the agency is charged to protect, then the FDA Science Board should mandate that the makeup of the FDA advisory committees not be dominated by those health care providers involved in the administration of the drugs to be considered.

However well-intended, drugs, including oxytocin, administered to the mother during labor and birth rapidly filter through the placental membrane and enter the blood and brain of the fetus in a matter of seconds or minutes. Once the infant is born and the cord is clamped, those drugs or their metabolites which are present in the newborn infant's blood and brain are essentially trapped in the infant's circulatory system for days or longer.

The FDA approved package inserts or labeling of most of the drugs commonly administered to women during labor note that the drugs can cause an increase in fetal cerebral spinal fluid pressure. What does this alteration mean to the subsequent neurologic development of the exposed offspring whose brains have been unduly compressed during labor as a result of artificially ruptured membranes, chemically intensified contractions, and/or skull fracture resulting from forceps or vacuum extraction of the baby's head?

The FDA Science Board must insist that the FDA disallow ambiguous wording in the drug labeling that implies that a drug is safe for a given condition when in fact the FDA has never required that a drug to be administered to a parturient must be proven safe for the baby.

I understand that the FDA uses its own definition of "Safe". But that is not the definition understood by the general public. To the vast majority of Americans, "Safe" means "free from harm or injury".

The FDA permits some pharmaceutical manufacturers to include in their labeling a statement which reads, in effect:
"Safe use in pregnancy, other than during labor and delivery, has not been established."
That is a statement that former Commissioner Schmidt might well have referred to as "weasel wording". Where is the documented scientific evidence that drugs such as bupivacaine, fentanyl and oxytocin are safe for the exposed fetus when used in obstetric care?

Research now suggests that oxytocin administered to the parturient during labor and birth may contribute to the incidence of autism in the exposed offspring. But is it the oxytocin that is causing the autism, or the epidural that frequently precipitates the need for oxytocin to stimulate the uterine musculature made ineffective by the bupivacaine?

It is ludicrous that scientists in the United States are still having to hash through the 40 year old Collaborative Perinatal Project to investigate the possible effect of obstetric drugs on human development. I have been told by several physicians who participated in that project that the Collaborative Project contained no control group of healthy, undrugged mothers and their babies who could have been used as controls against which to measure deviations from normal.

The FDA Science Board owes it to the American public to mandate that the FDA make every effort to require pharmaceutical manufacturers to document that their products will have no adverse effect on the immediate and long-term well-being of the children exposed to their products in utero, or provide with their products a package insert that clearly spells out the potential risks to the mother and her baby.

Industry must be reminded that they and the FDA are working in an electronic glass house. The FDA Science Board must urge the FDA to require more extensive evaluation when considering for approval a drug or device to be used in obstetric care. It is time that the FDA encourage manufacturers of drugs approved for use in obstetric care to submit data that demonstrates that the drug will not cause a delay in the newborn infant's time to sustained respiration, or interfere with the newborn infant's ability to see, to hear or suckle immediately after birth. Parents, as well as health care providers, need to be advised as to whether a drug will interfere with the newborn's normal ability to adapt to extrauterine life.

Concern regarding the long term effects of chemically altering brain chemistry was expressed two decades ago by Dr. Donald Towers, Director of the National Institute of Neurologic Disorders and Stroke, who cautioned:
"It is the biochemical circuitry - the biochemical messengers and relevant nerve cells in the brain - that form the basis for mankind's behavior"

Around the same time neurobiologist Joseph Altman, speaking at a Washington conference examining the possible precursors of learning disability, expressed concern that the development of the human brain appears to be programmed so that certain cells and nerve fibers must develop in synchrony, in order to make appropriate connections within the central nervous system. He cautioned that drug-induced alterations of the chemical components within the brain may interfere with the synchrony of cell and nerve fiber growth, causing subtle or gross misconnections within the developing brain circuitry.

The Neurologic and Adaptive Capacity Score (NACS), used in the past to assess the safety of obstetric drugs has been shown to be unreliable, and there is no documentation to support an Apgar score of 7 or above as indicating the baby has been unaffected by its mother's obstetric drugs. It is time for the FDA Science Board to develop its own neurologic assessment scale to evaluate the effect of obstetric related drugs on neurologic development. Even the leaders of the Society for Obstetric Anesthesia and Perinatology, of which I am a member, agree that the Brazelton Assessment Scale is the Cadillac of such assessment. The FDA assessment scale should be no less reliable.

As president or chair of several organizations concerned with the less than stellar quality of research in obstetric related drugs, I am here to ask why the FDA has shown so little interest in investigating the effects of obstetric related drugs on the development of the children exposed in utero to these drugs. In 1975, after the publication of The Cultural Warping of Childbirth, which I authored, I was invited to spend 3 months in a college of medicine, observing obstetric care in that highly regarded medical center. Since that time I have visited obstetric services in more than 70 countries and try to keep reasonably current on research dealing with obstetric drugs and procedures. I have found that there is very little effort to determine the adverse effects of commonly employed obstetric drugs and procedures.

I have organized and testified at two congressional hearings and instigated a GAO investigation, all of which pointed out the flaws in the testing of safety for obstetric drugs and devices, yet nothing seems to change. The FDA has not upgraded its "General Considerations for the Clinical evaluation of Drugs in Infants and Children" in more than a quarter century. And even the sound recommendations in that document have been ignored by the FDA advisory committees.

NORMAL PH DOESN'T MEAN OPTIMAL PH

A normal PH at birth does not mean that a newborn infant has come through unscathed. Animal research in New Zealand, carried out by Mallard and colleagues, investigated the neuronal effects of isolated and standardized brief periods of umbilical cord occlusion in utero. They found that brief periods of cord occlusion can cause neuronal damage in the offspring, mainly in the hippocampus region of the brain, with persistent functional changes in cortical activity, even though there was rapid recovery of other potential indicators of fetal asphyxia. Follow up of animals exposed to such brief periods of occlusion indicates that there is often a subsequent progressive decline in function. (Mallard EC, Gunn AJ, Williams CR, Johnston BM, Gluckman P: "Transient umbilical cord occlusion causes hippocampal damage in the fetal sheep" Am J Obstet Gynec 1992;157:1423-30.)

EPIDURAL ANESTHESIA AND CESAREAN SECTION

A randomized controlled prospective trial carried out by Thorp and colleagues has shown a ten fold increase in the rate of cesarean section among mothers who received a labor epidural. Separate investigations by Newton and others have shown that epidural analgesia can cause disruptions in normal uterine function that cannot be completely corrected by the use of oxytocin and can double the rate of stress incontinence.

Drug manufacturers would have you believe that the incidence and degree of toxicity of a drug depends only upon the procedure performed, the type and amount of drug used, and the technique of drug administration. What they fail to tell the provider is that gestational age, condition of the fetus, previous and concomitant exposure to other drugs, relative hypoxia and various pathological conditions can affect how a drug given to the mother will affect her fetus during labor, birth and the infant's development following birth. Hypoxemia and a resulting build up of lactic acid in the fetal blood during labor and birth can increase the uptake of a maternal drug by the fetal brain and heart.

EFFECT OF EPIDURAL ANESTHESIA ON NEWBORN

I suggest that before approving a drug for use in obstetric care that the FDA require an investigation into the potential of the drug to produce creatine phosphokinase (CPKs) in the blood of newborns 18 to 24 hours after birth. A study by neonatologist Susan Combs found a correlation between CPKs and CPK isoenzymes in the blood of the newborns who experienced asphyxia during labor. Increased creatine phosphokinase (CPK) and its isoenzymes reflect damage to cells caused by ischemia, hypoxia, trauma and metabolic disorders. CPK is found mainly in brain tissue, CPK in heart, and CPK in muscle. Her study underscores the need to use evidence of CPK and CPK isoenzymes as a measure of cellular damage in asphyxiated infants.

Combs found that those infants with moderate-severe fetal heart rate decelerations had chemical evidence of more cellular damage to brain and heart than to muscle compared to infants with normal FHR tracings or those with only mild variable decelerations. As decelerations worsened, a smaller percentage of total CPK arose from muscle and thus more from brain and heart. The data thus add further support to abnormal fetal heart rate patterns as an indicator of fetal asphyxia.

Research carried out by Stirrat and colleagues at the Bristol University in England has shown that an epidural disrupts the newborn's neurologic control of respiration for at least the first 48 to 72 hours after birth.

I have attended enough FDA advisory meetings to know that the questions posed to the new drug applicants are worded to avoid any implication that the baby may be adversely affected by the drug under deliberation. Some years ago neonatologist Jack Scanlon reminded the Society of Obstetric Anesthesiology and Perinatology (SOAP) that they were not actively looking for adverse fetal effects resulting from obstetric anesthesia. His ended his comments by saying,
"If you don't look, you wont find".

Again, I appreciate this opportunity to share my concerns with you. I have a very large collection of scientific papers dealing with the effects of obstetric drugs on the newborn and would be happy to share information with you. I am submitting a copy of the paper I presented for UNICEF in Thailand entitled *"DRUGS USED IN LABOR AND BIRTH: Their Effects on Mother and Baby"* and would welcome your constructive criticism and comments. Thank you for your attention.

Addendum: Nov.25, 2000
* The package insert must:
a) advise the reader that fetal hypoxia increases the transfer of most drugs from the maternal compartment to the fetal circulation.
b) define the FDA's version of Safe".
c) avoid the phrase "Safe use in pregnancy, other than in labor, has not been determined".

QUESTIONS OF DRUG SAFETY:
The FDA Science Board must develop standards for both maternal and fetal safety when the FDA is evaluating the potential risks versus the safety of any drug being considered for use in pregnancy or parturition.
DOES THE DRUG BEING EVALUATED BY THE FDA FOR SAFE USE IN PREGNANCY, PARTURITION, OR LACTATION INCREASE THE PARTURIENT'S :

- need for external or internal electronic fetal monitoring?
- disruption of her gag reflex?

- need for intravenous feeding?

- discomfort from pruritus?

- intrapartum and/or postpartum urinary retention requiring catheterization?

- the length of the first and second stage of labor?
- shoulder dystocia
- likelihood that she will experience an increase in internal temperature or a disruption in a) peripheral vascular tone, (b) normal thermoregulation, and/or (c) cardiac function?
- need for uterine stimulants, cervical ripeners or other drugs to counteract the effects of a previously administered drug.
- incidence of:

    a) disrupted internal temperature,

    b) disrupted peripheral vascular tone

    c) disrupted normal thermoregulation?

    d) anaphylactic reaction

    e) postpartum hemorrhage

    f) cardiac arrhythmias

    g) fatal afibrinogenenemia

    h) hypertensive episodes

    i) subarachnoid hemorrhage

    j) high or total spinal block

    k) brain embolism

    l) premature ventricular contraction

    m) pelvic hematoma

    n) uterine hypertonicity

    o) uterine spasm

    p) tetanic contractions

    q) nerve damage

r) uterine rupture

s) increased blood loss

t) headache and or backache

u) drug induced headache requiring blood patch

v) convulsions

w) aspiration of vomitus

x) coma

y) fatal oxytocin-induced water intoxication

z) subsequent fecal and urinary incontinence,

- inhibit the normal effectiveness of the pelvic musculature to rotate the fetus into the normal position for birth and expel the baby?
- inhibit the mother's normal expulsive efforts to bear down for birth, and to expel the placenta without the need for fundal pressure?
- persistent anesthesia and/or paresthesia (perverted sensation)
- weakness and/or paralysis of the lower extremities
- the need for fundal pressure?
- the need for an episiotomy?
- the incidence of 2nd, 3rd, and 4th degree tears resulting from extensions of parturients' episiotomy?
- the intensity, as well as the incidence, of postpartum hemorrhage?
- loss of sphincter control
- the incidence of central nervous system infection in the parturient or the newborn?
- the incidence of cesarean section
- the need for uterine stimulants to counteract the effects of the epidural or

other forms of pain relief)?

- the incidence of hysterectomy resulting from uterine rupture or infection due to cesarean section?

- loss of perineal sensation

- loss of sexual function

- septic meningitis or meningismus (symptoms, but without infection)

- cranial nerve palsies due to traction on nerves from loss of cerebrospinal fluid.

REGARDING THE DIRECT EFFECTS OF THE DRUG IN QUESTION ON THE FETUS OR NEWBORN INFANT: WILL THE ADMINISTRATION OF THIS DRUG TO THE PARTURIENT INCREASE THE INCIDENCE OF:

- non-normal fetal heart rates or tracings C fetal bradycardia, tachycardia or heart rate decelerations?

- premature ventricular contractions and other arrhythmias

- fetal-maternal transfusion?

- fetal asphyxia, hypoxia or fetal distress?

- meconium staining during parturition?

- meconium aspiration during parturition

- low 1 and 5 minute APGAR scores

- neonatal jaundice

- neonatal retinal hemorrhage

- permanent central nervous system or brain damage

- fetal death

- forceps extraction or vacuum extraction of the newborn

- nerve damage in the mother, fetus and newborn resulting from the extraction?

- a 1 minute and 5 minute APGAR score less than 7?
- newborn resuscitation?
- respiratory distress in the newborn infant?
- ability of the newborn to suckle
- delay or disrupt fetal or neonatal gut closure
- jaundice in the newborn
- fractured clavical, joint dislocation, damaged brachial plexus in the newborn
- RH incompatibility (due to fundal pressure or oxytocin)
- disruption of platelet aggregation in the blood of the newborn infant?
- the incidence of central nervous system infection in the newborn?
- intracranial pressure or skull trauma in the fetus?
- the incidence of hearing loss in the newborn
- the ability of the newborn infant to focus on and follow an 1/2 inch object held approximately 10 inches from his face. (Brackbill,Y)
- the incidence of retinal hemorrhage
- disruption of the normal visual acuity of the newborn?
- the incidence of tremors in the newborn during the first weeks or months of life?
- disrupt the myelination of the fetal and or newborn nerve fibers?
- alter the dendritic arborization within the brain of the newborn infant?
- interfere with the normal thermoregulation of the newborn infant? or the parturient?
- increase the incidence of creatine phosphokinase (CPK) and its isoenzymes in the blood of the newborn (CPK is found mainly in the brain; CPK in the heart, and CPK in muscle)?
- contribute to later cognitive and/or behavioral dysfunction?

REGARDING THE EFFECTS OF DEVICES SUCH AS ULTRASOUND ON THE MOTHER, FETUS AND NEWBORN:

- What is the immediate and long-term effect of diagnostic levels of ultrasound on:
    - fetal cells, especially those within the brain?

- the myelination of maternal and/or fetal nerve fibers?

- What federal agency regulates the safety of electronic fetal monitors currently being used and those under new device application?

- Does that agency regulate the inspection of such devices? If yes, how often?

- Do diagnostic levels of ultrasound adversely affect the long-term development of the parturient or the ova within her female fetus?

- What are the hazards of improperly functioning electronic fetal monitoring devices?

- Does the internal fetal monitor:
    a) interfere with uterine or placental function
    b) increase the incidence of infection in the parturient, fetus or newborn?

Thank you for this opportunity to express my concerns.

Doris Haire
The Bradley Method® Advanced Teacher Workshop
Washington, DC, October 25, 2013
Introduction by Marjorie Hathaway, AAHCC

We have created a new edition of Doris Haire's book *The Cultural Warping of Childbirth* originally published in 1977, updated with a talk she gave to the FDA Science Board in 2000. I have had her original book in my library for a long, long time. It was printed in 1977 and that's the problem. It's the date.1977 just sounds way too old. Not that there have been many changes in obstetrics. In the new edition we have put both talks together and added her talk today in a 2014 edition.

By way of introduction, Doris Haire is a medical sociologist with an honorary doctorate in medical science. Please look at the next to last pages of this book and you will see some of the amazing accomplishments she has initiated and accomplished in the field of childbirth awareness.

I cannot even remember childbirth without you, Doris. (Laugh.) We have known each other for a long, long time.

...I introduce to you Doris Haire.

DH: Thank you. I have known these two, Marjie and Jay Hathaway, seems like forever... I would like to thank all the husbands who are here. I first met Dr. Bradley at a talk in my home many years ago about Husband-Coached Childbirth. I can really see how husbands are important here today. (Applause.)

By the way, I brought my granddaughter who was born in my apartment in New York. All my grandchildren have been born at home and I'm very, very proud of her, I'm proud of their mothers, I'm proud of my grandchildren. There is nothing like a home birth experience.

I would like to start with a question. How many of you have ever heard of an obstetric drug advertised on television? Mentioned or defended? Epidurals, but never drugs. I am talking about drugs like they advertise other drugs like Pradaxa? There's a reason for that. They would have to provide information for informed consent. The pregnant patient has a right, prior to the administration of any drug or procedure to be informed by the health professional caring for her, of any potential direct and indirect effects, short or long term, risks or hazards to herself or her unborn baby or newborn infant which may result from the use of a drug or procedure prescribed for or administered to her during pregnancy, labor, birth and lactation.

My husband is a lawyer and was president of a hospital for 10 years and I can tell you, you are not going to get anybody to advertise an obstetric drug because they cannot admit that their product can be dangerous, and there are at least 3 maybe 4 groups of health professionals that don't want that information out. First of all are the obstetrician and the nurse. The nurse is the last one to be held as responsible as the person who is giving that drug. That came to me from Columbia University Medical Center so it's not just

Printed by permission of the Author Doris Haire ©2018 AAHCC

my attitude.

The thing that fascinates me is that one group that is so opposed to giving information for informed consent is lawyers. And I asked a few lawyers, why are you so opposed to informed consent? And they said because it makes it so much harder to sue the doctor or hospital.

As a member of the NIH data monitoring committee of obstetric pharmaceutical research, I attended a meeting at the National Institutes of Health. Two of the risk minimization tools discussed at that meeting were education and outreach, intended to inform patients about the products risk, and reminder systems to guide patients and health care providers in using products in a way that minimizes risk. The FDA approved labels which the public tends to refer to as the "package insert" as one of these key tools. In light of the fact that many makers of pregnancy related drugs have removed their labels from the Physicians' Desk Reference, it is essential that the package inserts of all FDA drugs should be made easily available on the internet.

Now I would love to have someone go to Bill Gates and say, you made a lot of money off the internet, how about you sponsoring patient access to medical records? You need to know that you can get your medical records, there is a way of doing everything, smiling, if you just learn the system. I am concerned that the combined agencies will fail to treat the fetus as an important, extremely vulnerable patient. I have just read the current label of nine of the twelve most common obstetric drugs that have been approved by the FDA for use in obstetrics. I am concerned that at a time when women are becoming more wary of the risks of obstetric drugs, The FDA has chosen to water down the information in the package inserts for those drugs. Until recently one could tell whether or not a drug had been specifically approved by the FDA for obstetric use by looking at the indications section of the package insert, a section near the front of the label. If an obstetric use was not mentioned in this section of the label, then the drug's use in obstetrics was identified as 'off-label'. Off-label is a concept whereby a medical doctor may use any drug approved by the FDA for any purpose they feel is appropriate, even if that drug is not approved for that purpose. Now the FDA is approving labeling that drops this reference and uses the word 'indications'. Well, what does indications really mean? Does it say safety? We need a very clear way of understanding the FDA.

Sorry, I sometimes get a little impassioned by this thing. Frankly I'm dead mad. Now the FDA is approving labelling that drops this reference as the indication section. The lack of the term is misleading because it obscures the difference between off-label and a use approved by the FDA. That watered down language appears in the latest Marcaine labeling and the labelling of Bupivacaine (generic form of Marcaine). I would like all of you to get a copy of the label for Marcaine. It is one of the most important drugs used in obstetrics. They have now got good research to show that Marcaine can cause, it is a big word, 'neural apoptosis'.

At the University of Virginia, I had a meeting with the doctor who did the research on this drug. She had been researching alcohol on an Indian reservation and she found a great deal of learning disability among Indian children. So she decided that she would look at other drugs that simulated or were close to the chemical composition of the drug Bupivacaine. And what she found was that neural apoptosis can occur. Most of the research that claims to prove safety was done on rats, at least the beginning research. She found that in pregnant and parturient rats when giving birth the drug (and also alcohol) can cause a programmed death of brain cells (neural apoptosis). Now, I think you should all learn the meaning of neural apoptosis, because it is a great way to start a conversation with the hospital.

The FDA has approved Marcaine in its generic form for use in obstetrics, even though the agency has classified it as a Category C drug. The FDA's interpretation of Category C is as follows: risk cannot be ruled out, adequate well-controlled human studies are lacking, and animal studies have shown risk to the fetus are lacking as well. There is a chance of fetal harm if the drug is administered during pregnancy, but the potential benefits may outweigh the potential risks. Now how can you outweigh potential risks if you don't know them?

Let's focus on the sentence: "… adequate and well controlled human studies are lacking, and animal studies have shown a risk to the fetus or are lacking as well…"

I have called several individuals' attention to the wording of that sentence, and no one seems to have been able to figure out what it means, even people in the industry cannot. In November of 2000 the science board of the FDA invited me to present my concerns regarding the safety standards of the FDA. Members of the science board did not challenge a single statement that I made during my presentation, nor during the following months while they reviewed the accuracy of my concerns. My concerns are nothing new. The 1975 FDA document entitled General Considerations for the Clinical Evaluation of Drugs in Infants was prepared by the American Academy of Pediatrics committee on the fetus and newborn. That document acknowledged that drugs trapped in the infant's brain at birth have the potential to adversely affect the rapidly developing nerve circuitry of the brain and central nervous system by altering the following: neuronal maturation (the rate at which the nerve cells in the brain mature); cell migration (the process by which the brain cells develop individual characteristics and capacity to carry out specific functions); dendritic arborization (the process by which the brain cells are guided into their proper place within the brain and central nervous system); cell migration (the interconnection of the branch-like nerve fibers as the circuitry of the brain is formed).

Dr. Caldeyro-Barcia was saying that Marcaine has the potential to dis-align how the brain connects, because some fibers in the brain are made slower than others by this drug. That is the way they feel this happens to ADHD kids, some can't read, some can't speak, some can't smile.

Now the work of Zheng, Heintz, and Hatten reaffirms that the migration of neurons along the glial fibers of the brain can be altered by changing the normal chemistry of the rapidly developing brain. At no other time in an individual's life is his or her brain more vulnerable to alteration, trauma or permanent injury than during the hours which surround the individual's birth. The nerve circuitry of the brain and central nervous system of the fetus is rapidly developing as the labor begins, making these complex fibers vulnerable to permanent alteration or damage from the drugs and procedures administered to the mother during that time. The FDA knows that none of the drugs used in obstetric care has been subjected to a properly controlled scientific study and found to be safe for the fetus exposed to the drugs while in utero.

In fact, this is a really important thing to know. In fact, the FDA has no written standards that must be met by pharmaceutical companies seeking approval of their product to be used in obstetrics. The only honest way to deal with this subject is to tell the reader (and this I think would help to protect every hospital and all medical personnel) there are no well controlled long-term follow-up studies on individuals who were exposed in utero to the effect of this drug (that means every drug, not just Marcaine). There may be delayed long-term adverse effects on the subsequent physical, neurological and mental development of the exposed offspring that cannot be determined at this time. While, if the FDA is charged with protecting the public from drug induced injury, why does the FDA allow the adverse effects of obstetric related drugs to be so far along in the text of the package insert that the information is likely never to be read?

I have been in hospitals where the interns could not get the package insert for the drugs they are using. How many of you have been able to get package inserts from your obstetric service? The pharmacist's version is edited, you can't be sure that you are reading what is truthful about the drug.

You need the package insert (label) that has the company's name at the top. They're up for grabs if they're not going to tell you the truth, and if they don't tell you anything.

Our high infant mortality rate isn't our only problem. Millions of children in the United States are suffering from neurologic disorders, autism, dyslexia, schizophrenia, and many other neurologic diseases. The list grows larger each day.

American families are becoming impatient with an FDA that yields to pressure from industry to dumb-down information in the package inserts of obstetric related drugs and allows manufacturers to methodically remove their labels from the Physician's Desk Reference (PDR). I used to have a label that was three feet long in two point print, got a lot of attention.

You can see that I get very impassioned about this, because concealing this information is needless. Women are smart enough to make up their minds. Their education is so much better today.

As pharmaceutical makers today remove their labels from the PDR it is essential that the FDA make all drug labeling easily available on the internet. Begin with the relatively few drugs approved for use in obstetrics. What can be more important than the drugs that are given to a pregnant woman? This will allow both the health care provider and the pregnant woman to weigh the information presented by the FDA before the laboring mother decides to take or forego the drug prescribed. The point of our concern is not that we tell the mother what drugs to take, but just be honest about what they are being offered.

At a consumer meeting at the FDA in the Nixon administration, the

Department of Health instigated consumer meetings, they were wonderful, people could come to these meetings. I had a good friend; he was the one who took all of the complaints from people. He only got a few, he wasn't overworked. People are very reluctant to report an adverse drug reaction. I served for three years on the National Children's Study which cost this country 3 billion dollars. Very few if any people understand the physiological mechanism of birth.

In the three years I was there the only thing I promoted is the 'time to sustained respiration'. The Apgar score has no scientific documentation whatsoever, because it has never questioned the time to sustained respiration. The brain is growing at the time it is born, it is growing before it is born, the first moments of life are extremely important. In the three years I served on their committee they would never allow 'time to sustained respiration' in the birth record.

Around the same time neurobiologist Joseph Allman, speaking at the Washington conference examining the possible precursors of learning disability expressed concern that the development of the human brain appears to be programmed so that certain cells and nerve fibers must be developed in synchrony in order to make appropriate connections for the central nervous system. He cautioned that drug induced alterations in the chemical components within the brain might interfere with the synchrony of the cell and nerve fiber growth, causing subtle or gross misconnections within the developing brain.

I want you to write down "neural apoptosis". It is the strongest word you can use in health care today. Neural meaning brain and apoptosis is the programmed death of brain cells.

Discussion . . .

DH: The pregnant patient has a right; (this is the law from William and Mary Law School). The pregnant patient has a right, prior to the administration of any drug or procedure to be informed by the health professional caring for her of any potential direct or indirect effects, risks or hazards to herself or her unborn baby which may result from the use of a drug or procedure prescribed for or administered to her during pregnancy, labor, birth or lactation.

It is a woman's choice, that is all I ask. Women would like to have research. The best research that is going on in our country as far as I'm concerned is going on at the University of Virginia, the scientist who was working with Indians. She decided to look at drugs that emulated the same type of effects as alcohol and got the same results. But she has never spoken publically, to my knowledge. It is hard on people to be brave and honest in health care. Because my husband is a lawyer and has been president of a hospital, I do get special privileges, here and there.

There is a second concern about this. If a drug has a recognized use during labor and delivery, whether or not the use is stated in the indications and uses section, this subsection must describe the available information about the effects of the drug on the mother and fetus, on the duration of the labor and delivery, on the possibility that forceps delivery or Cesarean section or other interventions or resuscitation of the newborn will be necessary, and the effects of the drug on the later growth, development and functional maturation of the child. If any information required under this subsection is unknown, it must be stated that the information is unknown. Now that is the law of the land, not just a Virginia law, but the law of the land.

Q: What were you reading from?

DH: William and Mary Journal of Women and the Law... but my husband who is a Harvard law guy says the same thing. It is extant, extant is a very handy word, it means it is for now.

Q: Speaking in general terms how can we teach our students who are not going to do the research themselves. Some of them are total research geeks, and some are not. There are so many care providers that I don't think they are intending to lie but they are constantly telling people epidurals don't hurt you, these drugs can't hurt you, they are not going to hurt your baby. How can we scare them enough without coming across as fear mongers?

DH: When you go to the hospital and they give you a consent form, write on the consent form; *"Neither I nor my baby shall be used as a research or teaching subject without my consent at the time."* Just let them know you are looking. That you are concerned and you are smart enough and you understand. This is a smart group of people, and most people are not going to know what you know. But, they need it.

Q: What do we do about these doctors who have websites that list the drugs that they say are safe?

DH: Just ask them for documentation, and documentation is not "this is my drug and I love it". You really need to see the package insert of every drug.

Q: The major problem is that doctors are looked at as authorities on the subject, and they are very quick to say something like "It is safe" and the mother doesn't understand. Obstetricians are looked at as the utmost authority on childbirth, and they will flat-out tell you "it is safe" and they won't go any further because the mothers don't know to ask any more, and they just take them at their word.

DH: You just have to get across to them that you cannot accept their word; they have never done the research. Even this woman who has done the research will not talk to people. We have a problem in people being able to speak out against the system.

Q: I think that is our biggest hurdle, as teachers, to get mothers to question authority.

MH: The Bradley Method® has a FaceBook page and we invite all of you to go out today or tomorrow and put some notes on it. In our Student Workbook we do have a quote from the American Academy of Pediatrics that says there is no drug whether prescription, over the counter, or food additive that has ever been proven safe for an unborn baby. That is in the Student Workbook. Pretty powerful? Yep.

Q: My quick comment is you are absolutely right about the PDR. I did an article on the epidural drugs and its causes and effects back in the early '90s on both the babies and the mothers. You know what, it has totally changed today you cannot find the same information in the PDR like you could then in the early '90s.

MH: Everyone should have an old edition of the PDR; it is amazing what is in there.

DH: I have them going back 20 years; I just emptied out one bookcase and said this is where the PDRs are. So they can't say that they didn't know, and that is the great tragedy, they have known for a long time, but they just find it difficult to tell the truth. And I will not trust something that comes from the drug store, unless it is the actual package insert from the company that makes the drug. Because the fact that the drug store tells you it is safe, just makes them feel good.

Q: I have a perspective on responding when a student says a doctor or nurse says a drug is safe. Perception of safety is somebody's opinion. You drove in your car here, you could say that that is safe, that is your opinion, that is your judgment of the benefits and the risks. And the same thing with using any drug, there are always risks. It was safe for you to drive in your car here today, but there were risks that you took.

MH: I think the problem that we are facing is that, yes, you have to weigh the risks and the benefits of all these drugs. The problem is not knowing the risks.

DH: They have them, but they may not show them. I have been in the delivery area and asked to see a package insert - they will not let you see it. One of the things that really bothered me is when I first called up my drug store when I first moved into New York, I asked for the package insert for I forgot which drug, but he practically fainted on the phone. Package inserts are really important, but only the drug company's package insert (label) assures you to some extent about the safety of that drug. Why should they tell you, on page seven, that if you give a drug like Marcaine there may be no recovery? Would you ever see that in a drug store package insert? So you need to know that the company's own honor (or whatever they call it) is involved. Again we are not trying to tell women not to take the drug, only to know about the risks and benefits of what you are taking.

Q: When you go into the hospital they have you sign all the forms which actually is that you have received information for informed consent, and you are agreeing that you are accepting everything that they are going to do to you there. How do you overcome that?

DH: I would write what I said: Neither I nor my baby will be used as a teaching or research subject without my informed consent at the time. Hospitals have lawyers to protect hospitals, not the patient.

Q: Any time they talk to you, any time they suggest something, ask them to write it on your record, it is amazing how often they don't want to do that.

DH: Remember the "time to sustained respiration" is the one thing that they fight most. Because how soon that baby breathes has a lot to do with its intellect.

MH: Thank you so much Doris.

The USA is in 30th Place in Infant Mortality (Death)

PEDIATRICS

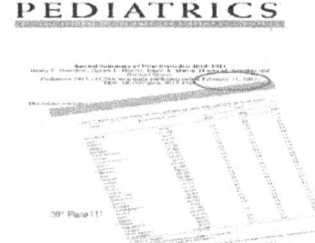

For more current information visit
www.aimsusa.org
or
BradleyBirth.com

PEDIATRICS
OFFICIAL JOURNAL OF THE AMERICAN ACADEMY OF PEDIATRICS

Pediatrics **March 1, 2013** vol. 131 no. 3 548-558
Annual Summary of Vital Statistics:

	Country	No. of Births in 2010[a]	IMR[b] 2010	2009	2008
1.	Hong Kong	82095[c]	—	1.7[a]	1.8[a]
2.	Japan	1071304	2.3	2.4	2.6
3.	Finland	60694	2.3	2.6	2.6
4.	Sweden	115641	2.5	2.5	2.5
5	Portugal	101381	2.5	3.6	3.3
6.	Czech Republic	117153	2.7	2.9	2.8
7.	Norway	61442	2.8	3.1	2.7
8.	Republic of Korea	470171	3.2	3.2	3.5
9.	Spain	485252	3.2	3.2	3.3
10.	Denmark	63411	3.4	3.1	4.0
11.	Germany	677947	3.4	3.5	3.5
12.	Italy	561944	3.4	3.9	3.3
13.	Belgium	129173	3.5	3.4	3.7
14.	France	802224	3.6	3.9	3.8
15.	Israel	166255	3.7	3.8	3.8
16.	Greece	114766	3.8	3.1	2.7
17.	Ireland	73724	3.8	3.2	3.8
18.	Netherlands	184397	3.8	3.8	3.8
19.	Switzerland	80290	3.8	4.3	4.0
20.	Austria	78742	3.9	3.8	3.7
21.	Australia	297903	4.1	4.3	4.1
22.	United Kingdom	807272	4.2	4.6	4.7
23.	Croatia	43361	4.4	5.3	4.5
24.	Cuba	127746	4.5[a]	4.8[a]	4.7[a]
25.	Canada	379373[c]	—	4.9[d]	5.1
26.	Poland	413300	5.0	5.6	5.6
27.	New Zealand	63897	—	5.2	5.0
28.	Hungary	90335	5.3	5.1	5.6
29.	Slovak Republic	60410	5.7	5.7	5.9
30.	**United States**	3999386[a]	6.1[e]	6.4[e]	6.6[e]

To be clear... the Lowest numbers in the right column is Best!

For more current information visit www.aimsusa.org
or
BradleyBirth.com

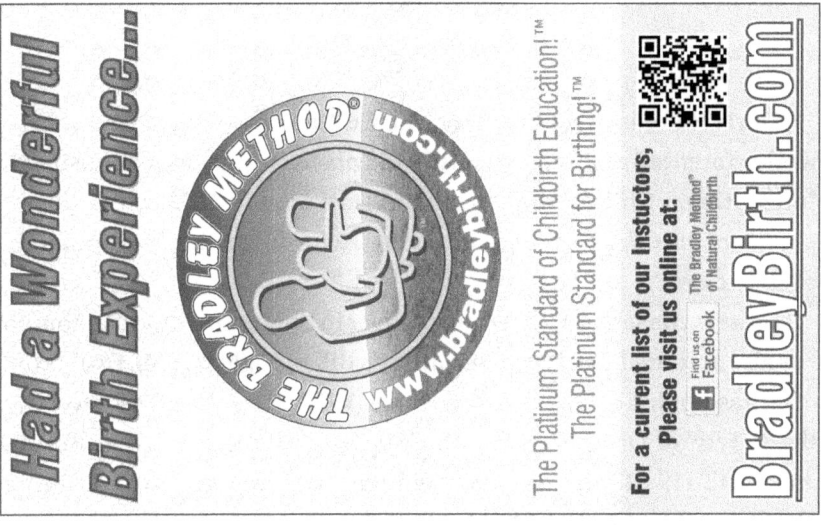

www.BradleyBirth.com

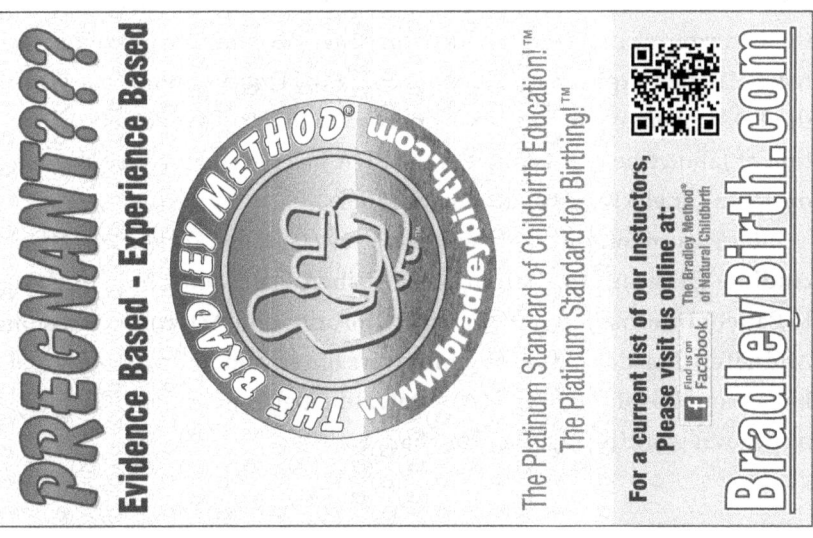

Doris Haire
...A Living Treasure!

Doris Haire is best known for The Cultural Warping of Childbirth, a well-referenced analysis of worldwide obstetric practices published by International Childbirth Education Association in 1972, while she was president of ICEA. This booklet marked a turning point in international obstetric care.

Haire, a consumer activist and pioneer in the area of informed consent, has also authored The Pregnant Patient's Bill of Rights (1974), Fetal Effects of Ultrasound: A Growing Controversy (1974), How the FDA Determines the 'Safety' of Drugs: Just How Safe is 'Safe' (1984), and Drugs in Labor and Birth (1987). She has observed obstetric care in 72 countries and continues to lecture worldwide.

At the invitation of the US Congress, Haire helped to plan and testified at three congressional hearings on obstetric care, and brought about the first General Accounting Office investigation into the FDA's questionable drug regulating practices. Subsequently, the FDA invited her to participate in a workshop held jointly by the FDA and the American Institute for Ultrasound in Medicine to determine information women should receive before exposure to ultrasound. Haire is most proud of convincing the FDA to remove the agency's approval of oxytocin for elective induction of labor. She points out that the FDA has never approved the use of oxytocin for elective stimulation of labor.

She was pivotal in the passage of several New York state laws including: Drug Information to be Furnished Expectant Mothers, Access to Patient Information Act, Maternity Information Act, and Professional Midwifery Practice Act, all of which were bitterly opposed by every major health and hospital group in the state. She believes in the effectiveness of women working together for change.

www.ingramcontent.com/pod-product-compliance
Lightning Source LLC
Chambersburg PA
CBHW070034040426
42333CB00040B/1677